COPING WITH BOWEL CANCER

DR TOM SMITH has been writing full time since 1977, after spending six years in general practice and seven years in medical research. He writes regularly for medical journals and magazines and has a weekly column in the *Bradford Telegraph and Argus*. He also broadcasts regularly for BBC Radio Scotland. His other books for Sheldon Press include *Heart Attacks: Prevent and Survive*, *Coping Successfully with Prostate Cancer* and *Overcoming Back Pain*.

D0730260

Overcoming Common Problems Series

Selected titles

A full list of titles is available from Sheldon Press,
36 Causton Street, London SW1P 4ST, and on our website at
www.sheldonpress.co.uk

Assertiveness: Step by Step
Dr Windy Dryden and Daniel Constantinou

Body Language at Work
Mary Hartley

The Cancer Guide for Men
Helen Beare and Neil Priddy

The Candida Diet Book
Karen Brody

The Chronic Fatigue Healing Diet
Christine Craggs-Hinton

Cider Vinegar
Margaret Hills

Comfort for Depression
Janet Horwood

Confidence Works
Gladeana McMahon

Coping Successfully with Hay Fever
Dr Robert Youngson

Coping Successfully with Pain
Neville Shone

Coping Successfully with Panic Attacks
Shirley Trickett

Coping Successfully with Prostate Cancer
Dr Tom Smith

Coping Successfully with Prostate Problems
Rosy Reynolds

Coping Successfully with RSI
Maggie Black and Penny Gray

Coping Successfully with Your Hiatus Hernia
Dr Tom Smith

Coping with Alopecia
Dr Nigel Hunt and Dr Sue McHale

Coping with Anxiety and Depression
Shirley Trickett

Coping with Blushing
Dr Robert Edelmann

Coping with Bronchitis and Emphysema
Dr Tom Smith

Coping with Candida
Shirley Trickett

Coping with Childhood Asthma
Jill Eckersley

Coping with Chronic Fatigue
Trudie Chalder

Coping with Coeliac Disease
Karen Brody

Coping with Cystitis
Caroline Clayton

Coping with Depression and Elation
Dr Patrick McKeon

Coping with Down's Syndrome
Fiona Marshall

Coping with Dyspraxia
Jill Eckersley

Coping with Eczema
Dr Robert Youngson

Coping with Endometriosis
Jo Mears

Coping with Epilepsy
Fiona Marshall and
Dr Pamela Crawford

Coping with Fibroids
Mary-Claire Mason

Coping with Gallstones
Dr Joan Gomez

Coping with Gout
Christine Craggs-Hinton

Coping with a Hernia
Dr David Delvin

Coping with Incontinence
Dr Joan Gomez

Coping with Long-Term Illness
Barbara Baker

Coping with the Menopause
Janet Horwood

Coping with a Mid-life Crisis
Derek Milne

Coping with Polycystic Ovary Syndrome
Christine Craggs-Hinton

Coping with Psoriasis
Professor Ronald Marks

Overcoming Common Problems Series

Overcoming Common Problems Series

Overcoming Common Problems

Coping with Bowel Cancer

Dr Tom Smith

PROPERTY OF
Baker College of Allen Park

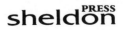

First published in Great Britain in 2005

Sheldon Press
36 Causton Street
London SW1P 4ST

Copyright © Dr Tom Smith 2005

All rights reserved. No part of this book may be reproduced
or transmitted in any form or by any means, electronic or
mechanical, including photocopying, recording, or by any
information storage and retrieval system, without permission
in writing from the publisher.

British Library Cataloguing-in-Publication Data

A catalogue record for this book is available from the British Library

ISBN 0–85969–929–3

1 3 5 7 9 10 8 6 4 2

Typeset by Deltatype Limited, Birkenhead, Merseyside
Printed in Great Britain by Ashford Colour Press

Contents

Introduction

A close relative by marriage asked me to see his mother, Sarah. I knew her well, but hadn't seen her for a few months. In her late sixties, Sarah had always been in good health. In fact, she had been a good athlete in her youth, and kept up her physical activities well into her sixties. For the last five years, sadly, she had had to look after her husband, who had been paralysed by a series of strokes, so Sarah was under some stress.

Even so, it was a surprise to be asked to see her, and she certainly didn't want to bother me. I had to drop in on her house unexpectedly, because she felt it an imposition for me to be brought in. She was that sort of woman, always caring for others, while taking her own good health almost for granted. She was 'too busy to be unwell' she said.

Yet unwell she was. For two months she had been feeling 'off colour'. She wasn't keeping up with her housework as well as she used to, and she was finding it harder to give her husband the care she wanted to give him. She was very tired a lot of the time, and a bit breathless. She hadn't weighed herself, but her clothes were a bit loose on her, and she thought she might have lost a stone or so.

I was shocked by her appearance. She looked gaunt and hollow-cheeked. I felt that she had lost a lot more than a stone, but didn't want to alarm her by weighing her. I asked her at length about how she felt, and whether she had noticed any symptoms that could help me pinpoint a diagnosis. There were none.

I asked her to lie on her bed – which she was slightly reluctant to do, as she still felt that she was wasting my time. I felt her abdomen, gently. She had two tender spots, one in the lower left corner, and the other just below the lower margin of her right ribs.

This worried me a lot. Over the years I have felt many abdomens and this combination of signs was ominous. I asked for her to see her own doctor the next day, and phoned him (he was well known to me) to warn him of my thoughts about her. He was surprised. He had not seen Sarah for years as a patient, although they had met socially from time to time. He had no idea that she had been feeling unwell.

He phoned me the next day. She had been sent to hospital for urgent investigations, and our suspicions that she had bowel cancer with secondary spread to the liver were quickly confirmed. It then turned out that she had had symptoms for much longer than she had admitted to either of us. There had been occasional bouts of diarrhoea with pains in the stomach, and the occasional bowel movement had been flecked with blood. She had put the first down to dietary indiscretions and the second to piles. She didn't dream that she could have anything else.

Sadly, Sarah's reluctance to see a doctor for herself was lethal. The cancer was too advanced, and she was too ill, for anything but tender loving care. Sarah died within three months of that first meeting in her bedroom. It was a peaceful end, managed without pain, and she had the love of her family around her when she died. But it might have been so different if she had thought of herself just a little more, and recognized the signs and symptoms for what they were.

So this book is dedicated to her. I can't emphasize strongly enough that Sarah's case is the exception, and the main purpose of this book is to try to ensure that this scenario isn't repeated. My aim is to try to teach people how to know when they need medical help and how to seek it. If you do this as soon as you have symptoms, your illness can usually be caught early enough to avoid an outcome such as Sarah's. Your diagnosis can be made at a time when the cancer can be treated and often cured. This book covers early diagnosis and how the illness can be managed at all stages. It is meant to reassure, not to frighten.

It is also dedicated to Jacob. He had had 'trouble with his bowels' since he was a child, with frequent bouts of colic from about the age of eight onwards. At fifteen, he was admitted to hospital with bleeding from his back passage. It was thought then that he might have Crohn's disease or ulcerative colitis, and that this would be a relatively routine admission. However, instead of the inflamed bowel wall that the specialist expected to see at his endoscopy, there were literally hundreds of small 'polyps' – small fleshy growths – hanging from it. One or two of them showed fresh bleeding. The bleeding was stopped, and as many polyps as possible were removed by the surgeon.

The stopping of the bleeding wasn't difficult, surgically. What *was* difficult was what to do next. Jacob was asked about his family. Had any of them had bowel disease? He didn't know, but his mother thought that her mother, who had died in her thirties, might have had it. In those days people didn't talk to their children about their illnesses, so she wasn't sure. A little research into old files and his grandmother's death certificate confirmed that colorectal cancer was her cause of death.

Jacob was asked to undergo genetic tests, and it was confirmed that he had a form of inherited 'polyposis' of the bowel. This meant he had a hundred per cent chance of developing bowel cancer by the time he reached his thirties. A complete colectomy was offered to him, and he accepted it, gratefully. He is now a fit and healthy young man in his late twenties.

The stories of Sarah and Jacob could not have been more different, with different presentations and very different results. Yet they are typical of the same disease – colorectal cancer.

A few years ago, writing a book for the general public on colorectal cancer would have been difficult – and trying to sell it would have been impossible. Cancer itself wasn't a subject that was openly discussed, and bowel problems were no matter for polite conversation or even for a serious discussion with family and friends. When people noticed problems with their bowels, they usually kept them to themselves. They waited until their symptoms were so obvious (and sometimes so socially unacceptable) that by the time they sought help, it was often too late for them to be cured. Even then, they didn't want to know about cancer. The diagnosis was hidden from them. Their doctors would skirt around the issue, preferring to use words like 'bowel inflammation' or 'bowel ulcers' or 'obstructions', rather than to present them with the truth. It led to deceit, mistrust and suspicion, rather than an open and realistic attitude to cancer and its treatment and outlook.

Working in family practice in the first few years of the twenty-first century, I'm glad to write that things have changed for the better. Many people are aware of the risks of bowel cancer. They know whether or not it 'runs in the family', and they are willing to discuss their own risks with their doctors. They visit their doctors early with their symptoms and, when they do, they are properly investigated. If a cancer is found, it is treated comprehensively, and cure rates are far higher than they were only a few years ago. Most important of all, people with this illness – and their relatives – are told what is happening to them and how the medical and nursing team can work with them to make the very best of their future.

The very good news about bowel cancer is that the numbers of people in Britain dying from it are plummeting. Between 1972 and 2002, deaths from bowel cancer in men have fallen by 27 per cent, and in women by 43 per cent. This is almost entirely because of earlier detection and more effective treatment of the disease (Kmietowicz, 2004, p. 303).

So this book is an optimistic one. It is for people who have just been told they have rectal or colon cancer (they are the two aspects of bowel cancer), and for their relatives. It is also for people who fear they may develop bowel cancer. Perhaps they have had one or more relatives with the disease, or they have one of the bowel conditions that predispose to bowel cancer. Among these conditions are 'familial adenomatous polyposis' (FAP), 'hereditary non-polyposis colorectal cancer' (HNPCC), ulcerative colitis and Crohn's disease. They, and the risks they pose for bowel cancer, are covered in this book.

But the book is also for everyone concerned with their long-term health. For, although many cases of bowel cancer arise in families afflicted with the conditions listed above, most still occur in people in whom it comes out of the blue, with no apparent reason, and no family history of the illness. Why this may happen, and how you may avoid being one of these people, is also discussed in the following pages.

1

Colorectal cancer – who gets it?

In every illness there is a debate about how much blame can be apportioned to nature (the patient's genetic background) and to nurture (the patient's lifestyle and eating habits). It is an important debate in colorectal cancer in particular, because there is evidence that even when our family history is against us, and there is a strong risk of cancer developing, how we live and eat, and what we can do to minimize the risk, makes a big difference.

One person in every 25 in Western countries such as Britain or the United States eventually develops colorectal cancer (the medical name for bowel cancer). Every year in Britain, it is newly diagnosed in 35,000 men and women, and around 18,000 die from it. Men seem to be slightly more at risk of rectal cancer, and women of colonic cancer (higher up the bowel). The risk of developing this illness rises steadily as we grow older, with the average age at which it is diagnosed being between 60 and 65.

What puts some people at higher risk than others? In the Introduction I mentioned that there are diseases that predispose to bowel cancer – FAP, HNPCC, ulcerative colitis and Crohn's disease being the main ones. However, people with these conditions only account for a small proportion of bowel cancer cases. Around 90 per cent of bowel cancers occur in people who have no history of the disease in their family. This confirms the strong medical suspicion that what we eat and how we live are at least as important as what we inherit.

There is good evidence to back this suspicion. For example, in southern European countries like Spain, Italy and Greece, far fewer cases of colorectal cancer are reported per head of population than in northern countries such as Germany and Britain. It is rare in Japan.

Researchers propose that there are two mechanisms working together to promote bowel cancer in northern Europeans and North Americans. The first relates to the type of fat we tend to eat. We eat more fats derived from land animals, and fewer vegetables and fruits, than do southern Europeans, Asians or Africans. Fats are broken down by bile (from the liver via the gallbladder) in the small intestine. Research suggests that cancer-inducing chemicals (known as 'carcinogens') may be formed by the action of bile on animal fats, whereas fats and oils derived from vegetable oils and fish don't pose the same risk. As these fats are the mainstay of the food in countries around the northern Mediterranean shores, it is no surprise that bowel cancer is much less common than in, for example, northern Europe.

The second mechanism for inducing colorectal cancer arises from our apparent distaste for fruit and vegetables. We not only don't eat the right types of fat or oil – we eat far too few vegetables and fruits. Eating plenty of them provides lots of fibre for the colon to 'grip on'. The more residue there is in the large bowel, the faster the contents flow through it, and the more often we open our bowels. This means that there is less time in each day for any carcinogens (derived mainly from those animal fats) to be in contact with the bowel wall. It follows that by eating plenty of fruit and vegetables we give ourselves a lower risk of any carcinogens in our diet causing colorectal cancer. A lifelong devotion to a high-fibre diet, cooking with olive oil, and plenty of fish, rather than red meats, can therefore considerably reduce your risk of developing colorectal cancer.

If there were any doubt about the fibre and colorectal cancer link, it was dispelled by Ulrika Peters and her colleagues at the US National Cancer Institute. They reported in the *Lancet* (Peters and colleagues, 2003, pp. 1491–5) a study of more than 37,000 apparently healthy people in a cancer screening programme. All had a sigmoidoscopy (examination of the sigmoid colon). The sigmoid colon is the last part of the large bowel, just before it becomes the rectum. It lies in the bottom left-hand corner of the abdomen, and is just out of reach of an examining finger. Of the 37,000 volunteers, 33,971 had no polyps, and 3,591 had at least one polyp in the lower half of the colon or rectum. The people who had eaten the most fibre (the top fifth for fruit and vegetable consumption) had a 27 per cent lower risk of having a polyp than those in the lowest fifth for fibre intake. The reduction in risk was greatest in those who ate plenty of grains, cereals and fruits.

That's why so many doctors don't like the Atkins diet that has become so popular in the last decade or so. It has been promoted so hard that the late Dr Atkins's book on his diet outsells world bestsellers such as J. K. Rowling's Harry Potter series and Tolkien's *The Lord of the Rings* – two books that sell in immense numbers because of the films made about them.

The Atkins diet instructs people to eat only foods that are high in protein and fat, and to avoid almost completely foods containing sugars or starches. This rules out all foods made from flour, potatoes, rice and most fruit and vegetables. The diet is decidedly low in fibre and, if the researchers are correct, puts the colon and rectal walls in direct contact with potentially very high levels of carcinogens. Most of today's doctors, myself among them, fear that our current Atkins dieters will be tomorrow's colorectal cancer sufferers. Devotees of the Atkins diet who shrug aside these fears should understand that it may take two or three decades for diagnosable cancers to develop after the bowel wall is first exposed to carcinogens. Not enough people have been on the Atkins diet for long enough yet to allay our fears.

Other aspects of our lifestyle have also been linked to colorectal cancer. The strongest link is with alcohol consumption. The more alcohol we drink, particularly beers, the higher is our risk of colorectal cancer. Why this is we still don't know. If you have missed the message that the safe upper limit to alcohol consumption is three standard drinks a day, you must have been living on another planet! Above that limit, we are inviting illness and an early death. One of the causes of the early deaths that forced doctors to publicize these guidelines is colorectal cancer.

On the other hand, taking aspirin regularly may protect us against colorectal cancer, for there is now good evidence from many studies that people who have been taking painkillers of the aspirin type (such as ibuprofen, sulindac, naproxen and indomethacin), say, for arthritis, have a very much reduced chance of developing colorectal cancer. The evidence is so good that people at higher than usual risk of this type of cancer are now advised by their consultants to take a single 300-milligram aspirin (one tablet of the adult-type aspirin) every day. The subject of aspirin and bowel cancer is so new and important that it deserves a chapter of its own.

3

2

Current thoughts on preventing bowel cancer – the aspirin link

On Monday, 10 November 2003, I reported on a medical conference in London on new approaches to cancer. It was co-chaired by Professor Nicholas Wright of the London School of Medicine and Dentistry, and by Professor Gordon McVie, Director of Cancer Intelligence, and Past Director General of Cancer Research UK. The journal *Cancer Futures* hails Professor McVie as the United Kingdom's chief advocate for cancer patients. One of his colleagues, Professor Chris Paraskeva of Bristol Medical School, spoke on the causes of, and possible new treatments for, colorectal cancer.

Professor Paraskeva has been Professor of Experimental Oncology and Director of Cancer Research UK's colorectal tumour biology research group since 1993. He was one of the first people to grow human bowel cancer cells, and he shares his expertise and his cultures of cells with everyone in his field of research.

His talk was an eye-opener. He was able, convincingly, to link the evidence of a dietary cause of colorectal cancer with the evidence of the ability of aspirin to protect against it. What follows here is a summary of what he said that day.

Because colorectal cancer is the second most common cause of cancer deaths in the United Kingdom and in much of the industrialized world, he said, there is an urgent need to develop new ways to prevent and treat it. As its incidence varies dramatically throughout the world, diet may play an important role in both causing and preventing it. For example, only 1.8 per 100,000 people in the subcontinent of India develop colorectal cancer each year. The corresponding figure for the United States is 34.1. However, as Indians emigrate to the United States, or adopt European eating habits in their own country (and as one who is besotted with Indian cuisine, I can't understand for the life of me why they should do this!), their risk of developing bowel cancer rises towards American levels.

Professor Paraskeva proposed that 50–70 per cent of all bowel cancers could be prevented, mainly by changing people's eating

4

habits. This would reduce the yearly numbers of bowel cancer deaths in the United Kingdom from 18,000 to 8,000. All that most people would need to do to lower their risk of cancer to a minimum is to eat plenty of vegetables and fruit. The guidelines suggest at least five portions per day, but more would be better.

Already, Professor Paraskeva said, we know a lot about the cancer-preventive effects of aspirin, vitamins and minerals, and the knowledge gained from studies of them should help doctors and nutritionists to persuade people to eat more appropriately. This largely means many more vegetables and fruit than most of us eat at the moment. I can hear you mutter at this point that you know all about the vitamins and minerals in the plants we use as food, but what has aspirin to do with this? Surely aspirin is a synthetic chemical, and not a normal constituent of food. That's true, but it's not the whole story.

What if aspirin were not a synthetic, but a type of vitamin, one obtained from plants which we need to keep ourselves healthy – without which we may be prone to diseases such as cancer, Alzheimer's and heart disease? This is not a fanciful question posed by cranks. It was seriously debated at the meeting in November 2003 by highly respected scientists and doctors at the top of their fields of research in Britain. Their papers concentrated on the effects of aspirin in preventing and treating cancers of several organs, including the bowel, cervix, breast and skin. But their debate led to a discussion of how aspirin might produce its beneficial effects – and the implications are astonishing.

At that meeting, Gareth Morgan of the Public Health Service in Wales proposed that aspirin may actually act like a vitamin. He has been studying the association between aspirin use and cancer, but he admitted that the link is not straightforward. Patients who take aspirin may be different and more health-conscious than those who don't, and early symptoms of cancer may induce people to take aspirin. However, the figures do strongly suggest that taking aspirin regularly can prevent several forms of cancer.

Mr Morgan summarized the knowledge so far gleaned from many studies. For example, a report on nearly 3,000 cases showed that aspirin substantially protects against ovarian cancer. For cancer of the oesophagus, the ninth commonest cancer in Britain, there are data on 2,000 cases. Taking aspirin regularly lowered the risk by half, a similar reduction to that for stomach cancer. Two studies of stomach cancer reported that the risk reduction was even greater in people whose stomachs are affected by the ulcer-inducing germ *Helicobacter pylori*. Even in lung cancer, four of the five studies suggest that there is a small benefit if smokers take aspirin. Aspirin use is also associated with a 50 per cent reduction in the risk of developing the skin cancer melanoma and the blood cancer leukaemia.

How could aspirin have all these beneficial effects? Mr Morgan's proposal, with which the rest of the speakers agreed, stems from an understanding of what salicylate does in the plant world. All plants, including vegetables and fruits, make salicylate in times of crisis – such as when they are wounded by grazing animals or are infected by plant-disease-causing viruses and fungi. Salicylate is part of the plant's healing process, healing wounds and killing infecting organisms. It is a mainstay of the plant's defences against disease. Could it be the same in humans? We do not make salicylate ourselves, but one reason we need to eat plants, Mr Morgan proposed, is to obtain the salicylate we need from them. Even carnivores such as big cats eat the small intestines of their prey first after a kill. This, it was proposed by the experts, may well be to ensure a plentiful supply of salicylate (from partly digested vegetable matter in the intestine) in their diet. Domestic cats and dogs eat grass from time to time, probably for the same reason.

Mr Morgan proposed that modern people are salicylate-deficient as a result of their lifestyles. They eat less fruit and vegetables than previous generations, and the fruit and vegetables they do eat contain less salicylate than before. This is partly because shops do not sell bruised or damaged vegetables or fruit. Naturally, salicylate levels are higher in such vegetables because the plant produces it in response to the damage. People were not so choosy in the past! Nor are they likely to go back to their old eating habits. So aspirin, acetyl salicylate, might well be a good substitute.

Not all the experts at the meeting thought it appropriate to classify salicylate as a vitamin, but there may be some sense in seeking a national health policy on aspirin. It reduces the risk of cardiovascular disease and is relatively safe in low doses. One proposal was that it might be taken from the age of 50 onwards by anyone judged to be at raised risk of heart disease or cancer, in much the same way as influenza vaccination is offered to people with lung diseases and other chronic illnesses. Mr Morgan asked the audience of cancer experts to start the debate, keeping in mind that wider aspirin use must be a complement to other health gains, and that its benefit should always be greater than its risk.

So it seems that aspirin may have a role to play in the future treatment of colorectal cancer, which I look at again in Chapters 10 and 11.

3

Your feelings and what you can do to help yourself

This book is largely about the way doctors treat colorectal cancer. Its main purpose is to help you understand your bowel in health and in disease, and how today's specialists can detect and treat cancer better than ever before. We are now in an age when we can do something for everyone who develops colorectal cancer, and the treatment of cancer has become a partnership involving doctors, nurses and patients. At every stage of the partnership, from the initial diagnosis through the difficult days of coming to terms with it, and through surgical and medical treatments, it is essential for you, the patient, to be wholly aware of what is happening and why. You have a say in what is to be done, and will take part in every decision to be made.

But how do you take that part, when you have just been faced with what must seem like a death sentence? Over many years of practice, like all other family doctors, I've seen people react in a number of different ways to the news that they have cancer. Many years ago, I decided to tell a minister of religion, who had been told by a previous doctor that he had 'severe ulcers in the bowel that would need many months of treatment', that he in fact had inoperable cancer and only a week or two to live. I thought that his faith would sustain him, and that it would help him to talk honestly about important things with his wife and family. The family themselves were in distress about keeping up with the lies they had been forced to tell.

In fact, telling him the truth was a disaster. He fell apart, and became hugely unhappy with his lot and with everyone around him, including his wife. He seemed to be hiding some guilty secret and was terrified of meeting his God. So now when I am faced with talking to someone about their cancer, what happened that day comes clearly into my mind. I am very conscious of the importance of delivering the news with sympathy and with hope, and to choose words that can help, rather than be brutally matter of fact.

The change is extremely difficult to accept. After a lifetime of seeing oneself as 'normal', it is very hard not to look on yourself as 'a cancer patient'. From receiving the news, you see your body as harbouring some malign influence that wishes to cause your death. You are now different from everyone else that you know, because you have this 'thing' inside you. It hurts emotionally much more than it hurts physically.

But you have to be able to deal with this feeling. You must not let it set you aside, in your own mind, from everyone you love and care for. You are no different from the person you were just a few minutes ago. You just happen to have been told you have an illness. The illness is not the essential you – the *you* that you always have been and always will be. You remain your usual self, with all your usual character traits and attitudes and feelings. You have not suddenly become an outcast from society or your family.

You will receive a lot of sympathy as a result of your diagnosis, although some people will be able to accept the news about you better than others. Some friends will rally round, and others will shy away – not because they don't feel for you, but because they don't know how to deal with the news. Cancer has a resonance different from other illnesses, even though today it can have a better outlook than other more 'acceptable' illnesses like heart failure or chronic obstructive lung disease – or even depression. So you can expect friends to react differently to your news. Often you may be the one doing the comforting, rather than being comforted.

Most people don't react like my minister friend. They take the news stoically, often hiding their feelings in front of family and friends. That's fine for a while, but it's good to let your feelings go once in a while. It's not wrong to cry or to show your emotions, and it often helps people to relate to you more closely. If you don't show your inner feelings from time to time, others may think you don't want *them* to either. That can lead to meaningless conversations and platitudes, rather than real communications and sharing of feelings. It is better that everyone knows what is happening to you so that you and they can understand and help in practical and emotional ways. Trying to hide the diagnosis from your nearest and dearest doesn't work, and eventually generates an atmosphere of mistrust.

On the other hand, this isn't the time to indulge in too much self-pity. There is no point in asking yourself 'Why me?' By the time you have cancer, it's not a 'why?' question. Feeling sorry for yourself all the time is a very destructive emotion: it takes all joy in life away, and drives a barrier between you and your family and friends. It can so easily slip into depression, and that isn't a mood in which you can deal with your cancer easily or effectively. Depression carries a higher mortality rate, in the long run, than colorectal cancer. Making the effort to be 'normal' in your relationships can actually lift your spirits. Humour is especially valuable, even when you least feel like it. Just because you have cancer is no reason to stop seeing your friends or going out and enjoying yourself. If you can look on your cancer as a temporary inconvenience, rather than a threat to your life, you and your family will cope better. In your darker moments you may not believe it, but your life can be normal again.

Of course, it's all very well for someone like me, who doesn't yet have cancer (as far as I know), to advise you how to behave. I can imagine as you read this that you will think, because I haven't experienced personally what you are going through, that I can't do so. That's partly true, but I can give from my own experience some examples of people I admired very much when it came to their diagnosis, and one of them is Jenny.

Jenny

One January, I had to tell Jenny, a young woman of 35, that she had inoperable ovarian cancer. It had spread from her ovaries into the liver and lungs. Being a midwife, she knew what that meant. She actually sympathized with *me*: her words were 'It must have been very hard for you to tell me that'. She continued by saying that she already knew that she had a terminal illness, and that she would do her best in the months she had left to make things as easy as possible for her parents, who were going to look after her.

In July that year I went back to that practice (I do a locum there three times a year), and was astonished to find that Jenny was not only still alive, but was well and undergoing weekly chemotherapy. That involves a round-trip of more than 400 miles every week, in her father's camper van. She was delighted to see me, but the best news of all was that the most accurate measure of the extent of her cancer had returned to normal levels. I'll explain this further.

In ovarian cancer we can measure how much active cancer a person has in the CA-125 antigen level. The normal level is under 40 units. That January, Jenny's first reading was over 1,000. After extensive chemotherapy in the spring, it had fallen to around 100. After another course in May, it had fallen to 38. She knows that this may not last, but she is enjoying her extra months – and perhaps years – of life. At the time of writing, she does not have detectable ovarian cancer on her scan and her CA-125 level is now down to 20 units.

Amazingly, she can laugh about herself and her problems with travelling so far for chemotherapy and how she has changed, both emotionally and physically. Anyone who visits her comes away from her room cheered up by her immense courage and humour and her determination not to make her friends and family, and her nurses and doctors, miserable. Yet I'm sure that there are times when, by herself, she is low and fearful.

She has ovarian cancer, a type of tumour that carries a far higher mortality than colorectal cancer. But she has all the qualities that can help her through her illness.

In fact, in my experience, far more people react like Jenny than like my minister friend. Something inside seems to help you face the problems in a calmer and more rational mood than you would expect. If you can cultivate that feeling, it will help a lot in tolerating your treatment in the months ahead. It will also let you examine your lifestyle and see how you can change it, if necessary, to give yourself the best chance of survival.

Healthy living and cancer

This is the one decision that you alone can make. To give yourself the best possible chance of long-term survival, you must live healthily. This doesn't mean becoming a vegetarian, following cranky diets, or taking vitamin and mineral supplements. None of these has ever been proven to prolong life once someone has developed cancer. In fact, some have been positively bad, as such diets often don't contain enough food and nutrients to maintain a normal weight or provide enough energy for everyday life.

The US Preventive Services Task Force, which advises the United States government, searched medical reports from 1966 to September 2001 on the use of vitamins in preventing and treating heart disease and cancer. They found no evidence that they were of any help in either case (*Annals of Internal Medicine*, 2003, pp. 56–70). Taking beta-carotene supplements, in fact, did patients with lung cancers more harm than good (*Annals of Internal Medicine*, 2003, pp. 51–5), and there is no reason to suppose they would help people with colorectal cancer.

So don't be persuaded by the many people who will say to you that they have a dietary way to deal with your cancer. It doesn't exist. It is particularly cruel to make such claims. No one can stick rigidly to such diets for a long period: it is inevitable you will backslide and revert, even if only for a short time, to your old habits. That makes you feel guilty that you are not doing as you were told. The people advising you will double this guilt by trying to make you believe that any recurrence of the cancer is due to your failure to follow their 'treatment'.

Do *not* let anyone do this to you. Many so-called 'health cure' promoters depend on this manipulation of your emotions and fears to make their profit. There is no place in cancer treatment for anyone who is pushing a programme of diets and dietary supplements for profit. And there is certainly no place for people who make claims that are not substantiated by facts that have been proven by unbiased statistical analysis.

If you have cancer it is very important that you eat enough of a wide variety of foods to replace the extra energy lost to the cancer cells and to supply the essential ingredients to maintain the immune system in its fight against them. In particular, the bowel needs vegetables and fruit to provide the right environment inside the colon to prevent the development of new tumours. The colon needs bulk to work on, which it gets from the fibre that vegetables and fruit provide. The natural salicylate that they also provide may well be a bonus, in that it may prevent the development of new polyps or stop them from becoming new cancers.

Your attitude

Peace of mind and the ability to relax are also a help. It is only natural to feel anxious and frightened when faced with the diagnosis of cancer, and you may well need help in getting over this initial phase. The medical teams either in the hospital or in your health centre will introduce you to professionals who can advise you. Relaxation classes can be a great boost, as can yoga classes.

It is good to keep up all your connections and relationships with good friends who are kindly and sympathetic without overdoing it. People who have just been told they have cancer tend to think they are now somehow different from the rest of the population. They are 'cancer patients' rather than normal human beings who happen to have cancer. You mustn't think like that. Instead, see yourself as the same person you were on the day before the diagnosis was made. It is just that you have this extra 'thing' that you have to deal with. It is not going to overshadow or rule your life. You can continue to do all the things you were doing before it happened to you.

Except for . . .

Well, all of them bar one or two – such as smoking. If you are a smoker, never light up another cigarette. You would be mad to continue to expose your bowel (or for that matter any other organ) to the cancer-inducing properties of the chemicals in cigarette smoke. If you are a heavy drinker, you should stop that too. A small drink every day isn't harmful, a night out on the tiles might be. Regular binge drinking at weekends is a definite disaster.

How to handle family reactions

You may have another problem – concerned relatives. If you have been told you have colorectal cancer, it is absolutely your right that this information be kept confidential to yourself and to whomever you choose to tell. Your relatives have no right to know anything you don't want them to know. So if you don't want to tell them, don't do so. Your doctor won't tell anyone else but you, and will leave it to you to decide who else needs to know. Naturally, most of the time it's better that your immediate family understands what is happening, so that you can all be open and truthful about things. But it's up to you, if you wish, to keep it from anyone who you feel would react badly to the news and who would cause you more stress by their over-reaction or excessive concern.

Don't worry about what your doctors might say to your relatives.

Even if your whole family puts pressure on your doctors to tell them your medical problems, they won't buckle under. They will support you in any instructions you give them about releasing information about your health. Doctors are often faced with angry relatives of cancer patients wishing to know more about the illness: we try to acknowledge, sympathize with, and understand their anger, but it won't make a jot of difference to our primary duty – which is to our patients. A prime part of that duty is to keep everything confidential between us and you, no matter how much pressure the family puts upon us. You can take your own time telling your family about your illness, and choose the people you feel you wish to tell.

A turning point in your life?

Many people who have just been told they have cancer have appreciated one other piece of advice. It is the perfect time to think about where you are going in life. You may find that the diagnosis of cancer is a turning point. You may change your job, review your relationships with your family, even move to that place in which you always wanted to live. It isn't right to make these decisions too quickly or without much thought, but often the decision to change is right. Perhaps work is too stressful and too demanding. Possibly you have been spending too little time with the children or your spouse. Perhaps you have put off that long-wished-for holiday for too long. Learning you have cancer concentrates your mind on the important things, and this may be the time to fulfil all those promises you made to yourself.

4

The normal bowel

If you wish to understand more about colorectal cancer, it's good to take some time to understand what the normal colon and rectum are, and what they do.

The colon is the last part of the gut, also known as the alimentary canal, the digestive tract or the gastro-enterological system (see the diagram on p. 19). That's why, when your GP wants to investigate your bowel further, you will be referred first of all to a gastro-enterologist. The colon takes the liquid content of the small intestine, made up of the remnants of food and the digestive juices poured into it by the stomach and small intestine, and dehydrates it. By the time it reaches the lowest end of the colon, its contents are fully formed into the familiar solid stools that we normally pass once a day in health. Just how it does this, and how the process can go wrong, needs to be explained before you can understand colorectal cancer.

The digestive process – mouth and stomach

The whole process of the digestion of food, then expulsion of waste matter, is a dynamic one. First the food, then the remnants of digestion, are propelled onwards from mouth to anus by co-ordinated movements of muscles in the oesophagus (gullet), then the stomach, passing onwards to the small intestine (ileum), then the large bowel (colon), and then to the rectum and anus. The co-ordination is controlled by messages from nerves inside the gut walls and by chemical 'messengers' secreted into the bloodstream by cells in the lining layers of the stomach and small bowel, in response to the appearance of food higher up. Sensitive tissues in the wall of the colon detect these messengers in the blood, and react to them by causing its muscles to contract. This pushes onwards the material inside it.

To start at the beginning: we take food or drink into our mouths, and with a conscious act we use the muscles in our throat to swallow it. From that moment onwards, we are relatively unaware, apart from noticing an occasional gurgle, of the food's progress through our gut

– until we feel the need to expel it from the rectum and anus perhaps a day later. Yet the gut is doing a lot of work to make sure we get the maximum benefit from what we have eaten.

You probably think that once we swallow something, it slips down into the stomach by gravity. Not so. As students we had a tutor who disproved this neatly by standing on his head and drinking a pint of beer upside down. He probably enjoyed the lecture more than we did! He didn't mind doing an encore either! It's unlikely that he would have been allowed to make such a demonstration today. Sadly, most medical students now learn from video presentations rather than from real, live lecturers.

His point was that food and drink get from the back of the mouth into the stomach by a ripple, like a wave, of muscular contractions of the oesophagus – the tube inside the chest that connects the throat to the stomach. These contractions push the food onwards regardless of the position of the person doing the swallowing. They certainly work in space, too, with no gravity. Astronauts have no trouble swallowing and digesting food.

From the oesophagus, the food enters the stomach, just under the diaphragm. The stomach is a very active organ, churning and mixing the food so that its surface comes into contact with every portion of it. In the stomach's surface are cells that secrete acid and other digestive juices that are poured over the food to start the process of digestion. The crucial part of this process is that the stomach only becomes active when it receives the appropriate messages to do so. This is where the principle that guides the whole digestive system in normal health comes in. That is, that what is happening higher up in the gut produces signals to the next part of the gut, lower down, to be ready for action.

For most of the day and night, the stomach is relatively inactive. Its muscles are relaxed, its secretory cells are producing very little digestive juice or acid, and there are only a few odd 'ripples'. But start to eat, or even begin to salivate at the thought of the next tasty meal, and chemical messengers are released from the mouth into the bloodstream to stir the stomach into action.

To put it simply, food in the mouth starts the stomach working. Food hitting the stomach 'kick starts' all the processes in the small bowel, and organs like the gallbladder and pancreas, that will complete the process of digestion.

The digestive process – colon and rectum

The same process – food reaching the stomach – sends off messages to the large bowel, the colon, to push its contents forwards to the rectum and anus, so that the stool can be expelled. This is called the gastro-colic reflex. Its purpose is simple: with more food in the stomach to be digested, the colon needs to be emptied to make room for it.

For most of the day, the rectum is usually empty. When we wake in the morning and eat breakfast, the chemical message from the stomach causes the left half of the colon to push any material inside it into the rectum. We feel that pressure inside the rectum, and have the desire to empty it. So we sit down – and, in the process, straighten out the angle between the rectum and the anus. The faeces can then enter the anus, and are expelled by our conscious use of the stomach wall muscles and internal muscles called the *levatores ani*. This process not only empties the anus, but all the faeces stored in the left half of the colon will be passed too.

Most of us in reasonable health pass around 150 to 300 millilitres of faeces each day. However, if we decide to refuse to obey the bowel's message that it wants to be emptied (sometimes the message comes at an awkward time), the rectum can expand to accommodate as much as 400 millilitres. It may even go 'into reverse' for a while, so that the faeces are driven back and upwards into the sigmoid colon. If we make a habit of doing this, the result is chronic constipation. It is best, if we can, to accede to our colon's first request.

The structure of the colon – its anatomy

The colon is 1.5 metres (nearly 5 feet) long, and is a closed tube. The small bowel, or ileum, empties into it through a valve (the 'ileocaecal valve'), so that once the food residue has passed from the small to the large bowel, it cannot pass backwards again.

It has four distinct parts. The first is the ascending colon that passes upwards from the lower right quarter of the abdomen to the area under the lower right ribs. It then turns a right angle to become the transverse colon, that runs from right to left across the upper abdomen. At the end of this second part of the colon it turns downwards, through another right angle, to become the descending colon, running down the left half of the abdomen. The final part of the colon is the 'sigmoid' (so named because of its resemblance to the Greek letter sigma – the equivalent to our letter 's') that lies in the pelvis, and leads to the rectum and anus. Where the sigmoid colon becomes the rectum there is another 'valve' or, to be more accurate, a 'sphincter', which holds the rectum and colon in place within the pelvis and contains some of the muscles we use in defaecation. At this point, for the first time since we had the food in our mouth, we become conscious of, and have control over, the contents of our gut.

The rectum then leads to the anus, the last 5 centimetres in men and 4 centimetres in women, of the gut. The distinction between rectum and anus is very important for people with colitis (about which more later), because the rectum is lined with glandular tissues, in contrast to the skin-like lining of the anus. As colitis is mainly a disease of glandular tissues this explains why the rectum can be affected, but the anus spared. It also explains why in colitis the rectum is much more prone to cancerous change than the anus.

Throughout its length, the colon is supplied with blood vessels and nerves that control and co-ordinate the work of the muscles and glands in its wall. In normal health, the colon dehydrates (removes water from) the liquid end-products of digestion that it receives from the small intestine or ileum. To do this it needs to have a normal layer of lining cells. These cells, collectively called the epithelium, work selectively to take back into the body large amounts of water, salts and minerals, while allowing the waste products to be concentrated into what we all know as a normal motion, or 'stool'. Muscle contractions in the colon wall push the drying motion onwards towards the rectum and anus.

The muscle contractions are co-ordinated by 'plexuses', or networks of nerves within the colonic walls. Electrical impulses generated by these plexuses cause the muscles from the ascending to the sigmoid colon to contract in sequence, so that the shift is almost always towards the rectum, from which the final fully formed stool can be expelled.

All these finely co-ordinated processes of nerves, muscles and chemical messengers working together are disrupted by the development of cancer. This is why the earliest sign of bowel cancer is often a subtle change in the normal bowel habit. It can be constipation or diarrhoea, or alternating bouts of both. It can also be bleeding. But there may be no obvious signs relating to bowel function at all. That's why everyone needs to know how to recognize the earliest signs, and what to do about them. As the main problems are often constipation or diarrhoea, the next two chapters will explain these things in some detail.

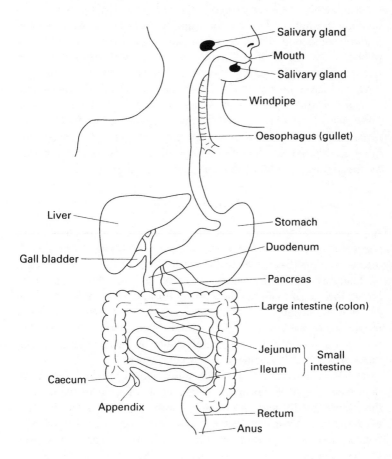

The digestive system

5

Constipation and diarrhoea

In animals and in primitive man – our ancestral hunter-gatherers of only a few thousand years ago – the call to empty the bowel was naturally followed by a moment's stop to do just that. We deposited a stool something like a cow pat, and then we walked on. Our progress towards civilized living, however, was the first step to abnormal bowel function. It became much more convenient to devote a particular time of day to a once-daily bowel evacuation. That meant training the body to ignore the 'call' after each meal. Most people settle for a motion just after breakfast. Because the faeces of modern man remains longer inside the colon, it became more dehydrated, and therefore less fluid. The cow pat was replaced by the sausage-like stool that most of us pass today.

Constipation

A once-a-day stool has become the norm, although it isn't necessarily 'normal' in the sense that it is physiologically correct. It means retaining the faeces inside the left half of the colon for up to 24 hours at a time. That's fine most of the time, but people who ignore their need to empty their bowel for much longer than that can get into the habit of chronic constipation. The longer the faeces remain inside the colon, the drier, and therefore harder, they become. It is then more difficult and uncomfortable, and even painful, to pass them when you do decide to open your bowel.

The Victorians saw this as unhealthy, which is why so many of their medicines were laxatives. Today we don't see constipation as a threat to health, and we aren't happy about regular laxative consumption. Most laxatives work by causing the bowel wall muscles to contract, so that they may even go into spasm or cramp, giving rise to colic. That's why many laxatives cause stomach pains, and people even judge them by the cramp they feel when they have 'a good clean out'. The older generation who grew up with daily laxatives being fed to them by their well-meaning but quite mistaken parents still feel a laxative isn't any good unless it causes a bit of stomach ache in the process.

In fact, the bowel gets used to daily laxatives, so that it eventually stops responding to the normal signals of a full rectum. A vicious circle starts, in which higher and higher doses of laxatives are taken: the end result is a flaccid bowel which is very difficult to empty. The only recourse is to stop the laxatives and try to re-educate the person into a more normal bowel habit.

Why do I bring this information here, in a book on colorectal cancer? Because the information we have gathered from the huge numbers of people with constipation over more than a hundred years has clearly refuted the most common misconception about the cause of bowel disease – that is, that so-called 'toxins' in the bowel, from germs in the contents of the gut, whether in the small or large bowel, are responsible for the inflammation that makes people so ill with bowel diseases such as cancer, ulcerative colitis or Crohn's disease.

In constipation, the germs inside the faeces are in much longer contact with the bowel wall, and are present in far greater numbers, than in people who have a regular once-daily motion. If germ-producing toxins were responsible for bowel disease, then people with constipation should surely have a far higher risk of developing it. Yet they don't. All that constipation causes is discomfort – it is not a cause of ill health. All that expense laid out by the famous (two recent royal ladies were apparently devotees) on regular colonic irrigation is for nothing. There is no need to irrigate the normal bowel: it is capable of evacuating itself, very efficiently.

Diarrhoea

This is where explaining bowel function in lay language becomes difficult. Having read so far, you could be forgiven for thinking that diarrhoea is just the opposite of constipation. In people with diarrhoea, you might think, the material that the colon collects from the small intestine has simply reached the rectum too quickly to be dehydrated enough, so you pass a loose stool. You would then follow up that logic with the conclusion that the colon is over-active, pushing its contents onwards too fast.

Sadly, the mechanism of diarrhoea isn't as simple as that. Diarrhoea is the main complaint of people with the two most common inflammatory bowel diseases: colitis and Crohn's disease. (The latter is named after Dr Burrill Crohn, of New York, who described it in 1931.) In fact, the colons of sufferers of these illnesses have almost no muscle activity. They are inactive, being flabby and almost inert. The colitic bowel is changed in a complex way.

To understand what is going on in the bowel with diarrhoea, we first have to define the term. That's not as easy as it seems. For example, most of us would agree that diarrhoea is opening the bowels more often than normal. But what is normal? For the hunter-gatherer mentioned above, it could be several soft stools a day. For most modern adults, normality is a stool once a day, usually after breakfast. Yet there are many who pass stools healthily twice a day or once every two days.

So diarrhoea relates to your own previous experience: if you are passing stools much more often than you are used to, you may be developing diarrhoea. However, if the stool is fully formed, and not runny, that may not be a true diarrhoea. The motion must also be looser – more watery – than before. The watery component is quite important. Irritable bowel syndrome (IBS) is a case in point. IBS is the most common condition for which people are sent to gastro-enterology clinics. People with it have bloating, pain and a changed bowel habit, but there is no structural disease in their gut. It is not linked to bowel cancer or one of the inflammatory bowel diseases such as Crohn's disease or ulcerative colitis. Many people with IBS describe what they pass as 'diarrhoea', when it is really a stream of tiny firm pellets, similar to rabbit droppings. This is not diarrhoea, and could even be interpreted as a form of constipation!

For the purposes of this book, therefore, diarrhoea means passing stools that are more watery than usual more often than usual. We have all had it. Most of us at some time have had gastro-enteritis – a bout of sickness and diarrhoea that has followed some dietary indiscretion. There are dozens of circumstances by which people can develop gastro-enteritis. Eating undercooked thawed-out frozen meat, particularly poultry or shellfish, is a common cause. Kitchen staff who are not fastidious enough about their hygiene is another.

Common to all these dining disasters is a germ that has been either inside the raw food, or has been smeared on it by dirty kitchen utensils or unwashed hands. If the process of cooking isn't complete, some of the germs are encouraged to multiply in the warmth, and they can then infect your gut in such numbers that they make you ill.

Understanding the processes that lead to diarrhoea is important in inflammatory disease of the bowel – and indirectly as to why it can lead to bowel cancer. Passing normal stools depends on the integrity – the good health – of the cells that form the inner lining of the gut. Their name as a tissue is the *epithelium*, and the cells themselves are *mucosal* cells – so called because they secrete mucus, the slimy liquid in which the digestive processes take place. Another word for the epithelium is the mucosa.

The mucosa, from the stomach to the anus, is a very active organ in its own right. It is the regulator of how much fluid we pass, eventually, in our stools. To understand why it is so crucial we need to know something of how it controls our fluid balance. So let's take a journey from mouth to anus, measuring the flow of water as we do so. The food we chew and send down to our stomachs is a semi-solid mass. The stomach adds a lot of acid juices, so that by the time it reaches the duodenum, the first part of the gut past the stomach, it is much more fluid, probably more than double the volume of food you have swallowed. You pass around 7 to 8 litres (12 to 14 pints) of fluid from your stomach into the duodenum in a normal day.

If you think this is a lot of fluid, then consider that to this volume is added juices entering the duodenum from the bile ducts (from the liver and gallbladder) to start the digestion of fats, and from the pancreas to continue the digestion of proteins and sugars. At the same time, the mucosal cells of the small intestine are pouring their mucus and watery juices into the cavity within the bowel. Doctors call this cavity, in which the fluid flows, the *lumen*. The volume of the material in your bowel lumen, by the time it gets to the end of the small intestine, and is ready to enter the colon through the ileocaecal valve, is around 10 to 15 litres (18 to 26 pints) a day.

However, this isn't just a passive flow of fluid from the mucosa into the small bowel. The mucosal cells are working hard, pumping exactly the correct concentrations of minerals (the technical term is *electrolytes*) such as sodium, potassium and chloride across their outer membranes – the surfaces that face the lumen in which are the bowel contents. In good health, the mucosal cells make sure that we get the balance of sodium and potassium, and water, in our bloodstream exactly right, within a very small margin. Recently we have discovered that zinc is also vital – but more about that later. To keep this balance so accurate, literally gallons of water pass in both directions across the mucosa, between your circulation and the contents of your bowel, every day.

23

You can see with an electron microscope the tiny gaps in the mucosal cell surface membranes (in effect, their walls) through which the electrolytes are pumped, along with the water in which they are dissolved. The chemical substances, or enzymes, produced either by the body itself in the normal process of digestion, or by invasive germs in infections, that 'open' and 'shut' these gaps, can be examined in detail. The technical details of how this can be done are well outside the remit of this book, but you can be assured that virtually everything is now known about how mucosal cells control the substances that pass through them, and what happens to them when things go wrong.

Infectious diarrhoea

A good example of that knowledge and how we have put it to excellent use is the modern treatment of cholera. Today we in the developed world look on it as a rather exotic tropical disease, and vaccination for it is one of the nuisances we must put up with when we are going on a tropical holiday. We couldn't be more wrong. In the mid-nineteenth century it was rife throughout Britain. People with cholera died from terrible diarrhoea until the public health authorities closed down all the sources of contaminated water and piped clean water to all our cities.

However, cholera is certainly not a disease of the past. It still affects millions of people in tropical and subtropical areas of the world where the water supply is poor, and people find it difficult, if not impossible, to follow all the good hygiene rules. I don't want to dwell on how people get infected with germs that cause diarrhoea, as this isn't what the book is about. However, what the cholera germ does to the mucosa of the small bowel is relevant to the processes that cause ulcerative colitis and Crohn's disease, both of which may predispose you to bowel cancer.

Cholera is spread by a bacterium called a *vibrio*. That's because it has a curly 'tail' when seen under a microscope, that vibrates to propel the germ forwards. Vibrios secrete from their surface a substance, which could be called an 'anti-enzyme', that 'blocks' – in other words, switches off – the mucosal cells' ability to suck water and electrolytes back through the bowel wall from the lumen into the bloodstream. So the normal two-way flow of water across the bowel wall becomes entirely one-way – from body fluids into the lumen.

If you consider that this flow can be around 20 to 30 litres (35 to

53 pints) in a day, you can see that the vibrio can create a tidal wave of fluid that has to be expelled as a mass of watery faeces. In a few hours, if that fluid is not replaced, the cholera victim simply dries up – that is, he or she becomes like a withered plant in dire need of extra water and electrolytes. Until we began to understand this process, cholera killed people simply by dehydrating them. Even when we gave antibiotics to kill off the cholera germ, it could take too long for the mucosal cells to recover, and its victims still died. Now we know better. Instead of dosing patients with antibiotics, in very severe cases we replace all the lost fluid very quickly by giving drips into the patients' veins. We let the body's own immune defences tackle the vibrio, and as long as we can keep the patient in good water and electrolyte balance, we can virtually guarantee a cure.

Cholera is the worst of the diarrhoeal infections, because its attack on the mucosa is so overwhelming. But the fact that even it can be controlled by rehydration – replacing the water and electrolytes lost in the diarrhoea – has established such fluid replacement as the main objective of all diarrhoeal illnesses. If we can keep the whole body's fluid balance correct, and take the stress off the bowel, it will usually heal itself. So when family doctors in Britain are faced with patients with the usual, much less severe, forms of diarrhoea due to gastro-enteritis, they normally give plenty of watery fluids along with the correct concentrations of glucose and electrolytes. If you have had travellers' diarrhoea in recent years, you will surely recognize trade names such as Rehydrat, Electrolade and Dioralyte – all powders that, when dissolved in a cup of water, provide just what is needed. The mucosa doesn't have to expend any energy to 'digest' them, and the cells can recover quickly. Meanwhile, the diarrhoea can continue until all the infecting germs are expelled. Once these germs have gone, the mucosa soon returns to normal, and the diarrhoea stops.

Today we hardly ever prescribe antibiotics or anti-diarrhoeal drugs for this form of diarrhoea. The antibiotics may lead to bacterial resistance, and anti-diarrhoeal drugs (like Lomotil or Imodium) may only prolong the infection. They may ease the diarrhoea, but make you feel a lot worse.

There are exceptions: typhoid fever is caused by a germ called *Salmonella typhi*. The cholera germ stays within the lumen and the gut mucosal cells. It doesn't stray beyond these limits. That's why we can safely allow it to run its course. But *Salmonella* doesn't stick to these limitations. While it initially causes severe diarrhoea and fever in the acute phase of the illness, it may also spread further, beyond the gut, into the bloodstream, and from there on into the gallbladder and kidneys. Once into the bloodstream it can cause overwhelming infection: the germs secrete poisons, or 'toxins', that can cause death in the acute phase. Prince Albert was one of its victims.

However, survivors of the initial typhoid infection may not get off lightly. The bacteria survive quietly, causing no problems, in the kidneys and gallbladder. Years after the original infection has settled and the person is apparently cured, living *Salmonella* bacteria can still be shed from the gallbladder into the faeces and from the kidney into the urine. These excretions are highly infectious, yet the person passing them feels perfectly well.

This is the *Salmonella* 'carrier state', and *Salmonella* carriers have been for hundreds of years the instigators of typhoid outbreaks throughout the world. The most famous was 'Typhoid Mary', who lived in the United States in the nineteenth century. Unfortunately, she tended to take work in kitchens, and moved on whenever an outbreak appeared around her. The story goes that she was identified and refused to stay away from food preparation: she did not believe that she could be responsible. Chased from state to state by the authorities, it is rumoured that she was eventually 'done away with'. She certainly disappeared from society in a mysterious way.

Typhoid fever is only one member of a family of *Salmonella* infections. Others include *Salmonella paratyphi* that causes paratyphoid fevers, which can be just as lethal, and *Salmonella typhimurium*, or mouse typhoid, which can also attack humans. All can turn their victims into carriers, so it is usual to treat them with the correct antibiotics that not only kill the germs in the gut, but also those that have lodged in the other organs. The drug of first choice nowadays is ciprofloxacin.

Salmonella was made famous throughout Britain, of course, when Edwina Currie, then a member of the government, claimed that most eggs and battery hens were infected with it. For telling what turned out later to be the truth, she lost her job and her future as a politician. It is still true that a substantial number of *Salmonella* infections are caught from eating poultry, either contaminated during slaughter or as it is being prepared in the kitchen, or because the poultry have been fed *Salmonella*-infected feed. Outbreaks of *Salmonella* have been traced to infected fishmeal from Peru, contaminated cocoa beans from West Africa (you don't want to know what was put on the fields as fertilizer!), and from seagulls depositing droppings on reservoirs after they have been visiting sewage works and landfill sites.

Salmonella has a cousin, *Shigella*, that is much less well known to the general public. *Shigella* is the cause of bacterial dysentery – dysentery being the medical word for extremely severe diarrhoea. It was named after the Japanese doctor, Dr Shiga, who in the 1890s first described it as a cause of an epidemic of illness in which a quarter of its victims died. *Shigella* shuns other animals: it is only found in the gut of apes, monkeys and man. And as few of us have close contact with our fellow primates, the only way we can catch it is to eat food that has been contaminated by someone who has been less than hygienic.

That isn't as easy as it sounds. When we eat a chicken contaminated with *Salmonella*, it is usually teeming with the germs. But they need to be present in their thousands for them to cause an illness. There are several reasons for this. One is that the stomach is a pretty hostile environment for bacteria. It is extremely acid, so that bacteria that can't tolerate acid too well die very quickly. The stomach juices also contain the very powerful protein-digesting juice, pepsin. The germs have to be protected against that too, or they will become just part of the food chain. After all, they are made of protein.

So when *Salmonella* invade us, they have to be present in reasonably large numbers, because only a small proportion of them survive the passage through the stomach. The ones that do make it through are probably protected by being thoroughly mixed with milk or masticated meat, so that they are not exposed to the destructive juices. But this isn't so for *Shigella* – these bacteria have a considerable advantage over *Salmonella*. They don't mind the acid environment. They survive the potential attack by pepsin. So you only need to swallow a few of them to develop a severe infection. A little lack of cleanliness after toileting, and your hands may have on their surface enough *Shigella* germs to make the clientele of a whole restaurant sick. When you hear of a cruise liner with a diarrhoea epidemic on board, or a plane in which half the passengers were ill, you can safely bet that it was a *Shigella* germ that got them. That brilliant scene in the spoof disaster movie *Airplane*, where all the pilots fell sick, was pretty close to the mark.

Shigella comes in two forms – *dysenteriae* and *sonnei*. The first was the one described by Dr Shiga; the second appeared later, and is less severe. But both cause fierce and very unpleasant diarrhoea that often needs emergency treatment, and that can lead to a form of true, lasting colitis. After a few days of watery diarrhoea and vomiting, the symptoms of *Shigella* infection change. The vomiting stops, and you start to have bouts of colic. These are sudden cramps, deep inside the abdomen and rectum, that you find easiest to relieve by passing, many times a day, a small motion that is less watery, but streaked with blood.

This is a sign that the germ has passed from the small bowel to the colon, where it has started to infect the mucosal cells. The bleeding comes from many small ulcers – patches of raw mucosa that have been stripped of its lining, epithelial cells, by the infection. In effect, the *Shigella* infection has caused an acute colitis virtually identical to the condition seen in ulcerative colitis, about which you will read more later.

Then there is *E. coli*. The *E.* stands for *Escherichia*, after Dr Escherich, the German doctor who discovered it. When I was learning bacteriology as a medical student, *E. coli* was accepted as a normal constituent of the colon, of humans and cows. It is only in recent years that we have recognized that some strains of it are far from benign. People have died from it in outbreaks of food poisoning, in which the beef responsible was contaminated at the abattoir – by careless removal of the animal's internal organs. The worst of these outbreaks was in the 1990s, in Wishaw, in Scotland, where the outbreak was traced to contaminated beef, in which the same cutting utensils had been used for raw and cooked meats.

The lethal form of *E. coli* has a different approach to infection from those of cholera and typhoid. It doesn't travel beyond the gut wall, but it has two unpleasant properties. The first is that it has found a way to stick to the surface of the mucosal cells. That protects it from being washed away in the diarrhoea it causes. The second is that, once stuck to the cells, it produces toxins to destroy the cells, so that they can use the residues of the dead cells as nutrients on which they can thrive and multiply. Once they have started to multiply, they quickly spread throughout the bowel, stripping more mucosa from it. The toxins can now pass easily through the areas of denuded lining into the bloodstream, from where they cause serious damage to the kidneys, brain and other organs.

A less common, but particularly important, diarrhoea-causing bacterium is called *Yersinia enterolytica*. Its importance lies in the fact that it seems to restrict itself to infecting a short area of small intestine just above the ileo-caecal valve, giving rise to a condition known as terminal ileitis. The 'terminal' here refers to the final part of the ileum, and not to the fact that the illness might be terminal! As Crohn's disease usually starts at precisely this part of the gut, and may even be limited to it, a *Yersinia* infection can easily be mistaken for Crohn's disease. That is a serious mistake, because *Yersinia* (but not Crohn's) is curable with the appropriate antibiotic. It is vital, when dealing with a bloody diarrhoea, not to miss an easily treatable condition.

So far, all the germs mentioned here have been bacteria, but they are only part of this complex story. We haven't started yet on the other infections that cause diarrhoea – protozoa and viruses. Protozoa are single-celled parasites, prototype animals, that infect other animals by getting into their tissues. Probably the best known of them is the malaria parasite, plasmodium, that in its various forms causes the four main types of malaria. Plasmodia are injected under the skin by mosquito bites, and target the red blood cells, and their life-cycle within us from then on causes the disease that has killed more human beings than any other.

Less well publicized are the amoebae, similar single-celled organisms that inhabit water. Generations of biology students in British schools have studied pools of pond-water and been fascinated by the free-living amoebae they can see under the high-power lens of their microscopes. Those amoebae are usually benign, but they have much less benign relatives that we call *Entamoebae histolytica*. They, like *Shigella*, can manage to pass unscathed through the acid stomach environment.

'Ento' refers to the fact that the amoeba flourish inside an animal's (i.e. our) gut. The prefix 'histo' refers to cells (histology is the microscopic study of cells), and 'lysis' is the dissolving away of cells. So from the name it is fairly easy to deduce that the main property of *Entamoeba histolytica* is its ability to dissolve away the human cells with which it comes into contact. In our gut, these are our mucosa cells. So the first achievement of an *Entamoeba* infection is to remove from the gut lining an area of mucosa – causing an ulcer.

This isn't all. Once safely ensconced in the small bowel wall, the

PROPERTY OF

Baker College of Allen Park

Entamoeba uses the nutrients it gets from our dying cells first to multiply like fury, then to create a protective skin around the 'daughter' cells, stopping us from digesting them. They can then safely travel further down the gut to the colon, where they then create havoc. The whole surface of the colon becomes infected and ulcerated, producing a bloody diarrhoea, and making the unfortunate victim very ill. This is amoebic dysentery, and is still a major cause of death in countries where the water supply is not clean, or the basic rules of hygiene are not kept.

Another protozoon, *Giardia lamblia*, is a particular favourite of medical students. With a heart-shaped body and a few wispy 'hairs' projecting from its rear, it looks under the microscope just like a tiny face. It's not so funny if you swallow it in your drinking water, however. It has a predilection for the upper part of the small intestine, from where it can cause a very troublesome, and sometimes bloody, diarrhoea. It used to be confined mainly to Scandinavia and to the countries of the old Soviet Union, but in recent years it has spread as people have travelled. The main source used to be raw fish, a delicacy in some northern countries that is probably best avoided unless you can be sure that the fish is parasite-free. Marination may not kill parasites in fish flesh: adequate cooking always does.

As for viruses, not a year passes without researchers discovering yet another virus infection that causes diarrhoea. Viruses, of course, are much smaller than bacteria, and are not seen with conventional light microscopes. They need to be inside a living host cell to survive and multiply. Only a generation ago, when I and my contemporaries were training as doctors, viruses weren't thought to be a cause of diarrhoea. We knew they caused colds: in fact, we knew of dozens of families of viruses that caused colds. We knew that viruses caused diseases like smallpox, chickenpox, herpes, hepatitis and types of meningitis, but we shunned the diagnosis of 'gastric flu' because we thought that viruses didn't cause gut infections. However, we couldn't have been more wrong, and around 1973 we learned about *rotaviruses*. They turned out to be the cause of the most common outbreaks of diarrhoea in babies' wards and nurseries in hospitals. Adults are less susceptible to rotavirus infections, probably because we became immune to infections with them in childhood. So rotaviruses are not seen as an important cause of acute colitis in adults. However, these viruses were a pointer to the fact that there might be many more viruses that could inflame the gut – and so it proved. Winter epidemics of 'gastric flu' may well be just that – a flu-like virus infection that is transferred not from swallowing contaminated food, but by being breathed in from coughs and sneezes.

Although we don't yet know the details of all the viruses that can cause diarrhoea, we do know what happens to the bowel when they attack. Bowel mucosa biopsies taken from patients during outbreaks show that the mucosal cells are abnormal: they have stopped producing their digestive enzymes and mucus. The result is that most of the sugar and fats in the food, plus a whole lot of water, remains to be passed on into the colon. The 'osmotic' pressure that the food residue of fatty acids and glucose exerts in the lumen sucks even more fluid from the circulation. The colon cannot perform its main function of dehydrating its contents, and the inevitable result is diarrhoea.

Where the viruses lodge in the intestine is difficult to pinpoint, but they are probably hidden within the mucosa of the first few feet of the small intestine, the upper part of the ileum. What we do know about viruses in general is that they do their damage by entering the cells themselves, and multiplying there, after which they spread to infect the neighbouring cells. They do not produce a long-lasting toxin. Once your body's immune system has got rid of them, the diarrhoea recovers.

Virus gastro-enteritis is probably the cause of many cases of travellers' diarrhoea. If you have had this on holiday, you will know from bitter experience that it can lay you flat for two or three days. Your only wish is to be near a toilet, and to have as much water as you can to drink, to replenish the fluid that you have lost. The best way to manage it is to keep drinking safe water and to add to it the glucose and minerals mentioned above several times a day.

Antibiotics are not recommended unless the condition continues past the first two days, or becomes serious and there is a suspicion of *Salmonella* or a similar severe infection. Antibiotics do not work against viruses and, as mentioned above, if it is another bacterium, you may just induce resistance, and become a carrier, if you take the wrong dose or the wrong antibiotic. If you have a lot of colicky pain with the diarrhoea, there is a case for taking drugs that will ease the spasm in the gut. The two most usual are diphenoxylate (Lomotil) and loperamide (Imodium). Many people take antibiotics or an anti-spasm drug routinely on holiday on the assumption that it will prevent travellers' diarrhoea. Neither will do that: there is no case for taking preventive medicines against it.

Diarrhoea in people who have had chronic inflammatory bowel disease

In the last few pages I have deliberately spent a lot of time describing the mechanisms of constipation and diarrhoea. I don't apologize for this, because the onset of constipation and/or diarrhoea in someone who has always had a 'normal' bowel habit can be the first sign of colorectal cancer. It may also be a first sign of the inflammatory bowel diseases ulcerative colitis and Crohn's disease, both of which are linked, eventually, to a raised risk of colorectal cancer. So if you have either of these diseases, you should be aware of that raised risk, and attend for regular follow-up accordingly.

We have established that any assault (as with an infection or inflammation) on the colonic mucosa will lead to looser motions. What is important is that such changes are recognized and investigated, and not simply left to 'go away' on their own. The next chapter will describe from actual cases all the common presentations of colorectal cancer, so that you can compare them with your experience, but I'd like to digress for the moment to the two main diseases of bowel inflammation that can lead to cancer.

The symptoms of ulcerative colitis and Crohn's disease – usually repeated bouts of diarrhoea containing blood and mucus – are very similar to those of infectious diseases of the bowel. Acute Crohn's disease can easily mimic cholera, and *Shigella* can easily be mistaken for acute ulcerative colitis. The diseases are so similar in the way they affect people that past generations of doctors were convinced that both types of colitis were in fact infections from an as yet unknown germ, virus, bacterium or protozoon. Crohn's was compared even with tuberculosis of the bowel, a disease that has thankfully become much rarer since all milk is pasteurized.

However, none of these searches for an infectious cause of colitis has ever been successful. That's a pity, because it would make treatment so much easier. It is curious, too, because the mucosal cells (see the last chapter) in colitis often look just like the mucosa in a proven infection, like amoebic dysentery. What is certain is that the mucosa in colitis is the tissue that is affected, and that it is inflamed and damaged, even if not infected by any outside organism.

Perhaps this is the point at which we should consider the mucosa in a little more detail. In health, the cells in the mucosa of the small intestine, as mentioned in the last chapter, must secrete mucus and be extremely active in pumping water and digested foodstuffs (the remnants of fats, proteins, sugars and starches, minerals and vitamins) across the barrier between the lumen and the body's internal circulation.

To do that, the cells are arranged in columns, several deep, and the mucosa itself is arranged in a myriad of folds and 'crypts' that are always moving and changing in shape. The constant movement and rippling ensures the maximum of contact between the contents in the lumen and the surface of the mucosal cells. If anything happens to decrease that contact between contents and the healthy cells in the bowel surface, then water will remain inside the lumen, and diarrhoea will surely follow.

The invention of the flexible fibre-optic endoscope lets us see exactly what is happening in all forms of bowel disease – and has been a huge boost to our knowledge of inflammatory bowel disease and cancer and how they can be treated. Using endoscopy from above to look at the stomach and small bowel, and endoscopy from below to see the colon, specialist gastro-enterologists and their surgical colleagues (they call themselves 'digestive endoscopists') are now able to see exactly what is happening in the chronically inflamed bowel and in the bowel suspected of being affected by cancer.

They make their diagnoses in two ways. What they see in the bowel wall is often enough to help them make a provisional diagnosis, and the microscopic appearance of tiny pieces of tissue (biopsies) taken from the mucosa usually confirms their suspicions.

The normal bowel looks obviously healthy through the endoscope. What the endoscopist sees is the inner lining surface of the epithelium – the mucosal surface. It looks unbroken, glistening, smooth, with the odd blood vessel coursing along it. The folds, ridges and valleys are easily seen, and there is the occasional movement and ripple as the normal muscle movement in the wall carries on.

In inflammatory bowel disease the picture is very different. In Crohn's disease of the ileum there are patches of red, swollen mucosa, with obvious ulcers (breaks in the mucosal surface, much like large mouth ulcers) in the patches. Between the patches, the rest of the bowel usually looks normal. The most usual area to be affected is the last few inches of the small bowel and the first part of the ascending colon, or the caecum. In some cases of Crohn's, the inflamed patches are also present in the rest of the colon, so that it is justifiable to call Crohn's disease a 'colitis' even though it largely affects the ileum, or small bowel.

Ulcerative colitis usually affects a different area of bowel from Crohn's. It does not spread into the small bowel, being confined to the colon. It tends first to affect the rectum and margin of the anus, where it is called proctitis, and then spreads upwards to the rest of the colon.

The two types of colitis differ in the extent to which they affect the bowel wall. While ulcerative colitis confines itself to attacking only the mucosa, leaving the outer layers of the bowel wall intact, Crohn's affects the whole thickness of the bowel wall. This can often lead to *fissures* (cracks that extend through the wall of the bowel) and *granulomas*, which are masses of chronically inflamed tissue, much like internal boils. The experienced endoscopist can quickly tell the difference between the two through the endoscope, but will still depend on the pathologist's report of the extent and severity of the inflammation before making the final decision on diagnosis.

Of course, not all that seems to be Crohn's or ulcerative colitis is necessarily one of them. Endoscopists have been caught by surprise, when what they thought before the examination to be a straightforward case has turned out to be much more complex. The biopsy may show an unexpected infection, or a rare type of bowel problem that mimics colitis. It may show the changes of cancer, either in patches of the bowel affected by Crohn's or ulcerative colitis, or as a completely separate disease in the bowel. That bowel may have 'grown' polyps or the cancer may have developed in a previously normal-looking area of bowel wall. Whatever the cause, the symptoms that have led the person to the endoscopy theatre are often the same. It can't be assumed that the onset of diarrhoea is always an infection, or even just another bout of colitis.

Looking back over many years of general practice and with some experience in research into gastro-enterology, I can remember many people whose first symptoms of bowel cancer fitted the classical picture, and a few who did not. They are described in the next chapter.

6

Some case histories

When the first sign is bleeding

I suppose every doctor remembers his first case of cancer as a student. I certainly do.

James

James was 59, and he was attending the outpatient clinic of our Professor of Surgery. We were both apprehensive – he because he was worried about his symptoms, and I because it was my first day of clinical medicine after passing my anatomy and physiology examinations. I was given five minutes to take James's history before I had to suggest what more I must do to make the diagnosis.

James was very kind to me. He knew it was my first day 'on the wards', and made it easy. 'I've been bleeding from my back passage, and I thought it was just piles, so I didn't bother the doctor.'

'When did you first notice the bleeding?' I asked.

'Around six months ago,' he replied. 'But it wasn't much – just a spot on the toilet paper, once in a while. I thought I had just been a bit rough on my skin when wiping myself. It wasn't until about a month ago that I noticed it every time I opened my bowels. Then I knew I had to do something about it. Even then I thought it would just be piles. I mean, everyone has that sometime in their lives, don't they? Even then it took some persuading from my wife to get me to see the doctor. I just wanted to buy some pile ointment from the chemist. The doctor found I didn't have piles, and sent me here urgently. I've probably got cancer, but nobody will tell me straight out.'

The conversation that followed was what nowadays would be called 'structured'. That is, the questions I asked him followed a strict order, something third-year medical students were trained to do in the weeks before they were deemed fit enough to see patients. I asked directly about his symptom of bleeding. Was the blood red and fresh, or darker? Was it mixed in with the stool or just on the surface? Was there more blood than initially, or just about the same amount? And how was his weight? Had he gained or lost recently, or was his weight roughly the same?

All these questions had a purpose. Red fresh blood suggests bleeding from the anal edge or just above, perhaps at the junction of the end of the colon and the rectum. Darker blood suggests bleeding from further up the colon. The longer blood has been lying in the bowel, the darker it becomes. Blood that has come all the way down the small and large bowel from the stomach, for example, is black, like tar. Often it is so changed that the patient does not recognize it as blood.

In James's case, the blood was red and mixed into the substance of the stool, rather than on the surface. That suggested bleeding at least in the rectum itself, rather than from piles, which are in the anal canal, the last inch and a half of the bowel. Bleeding from piles starts as the motion is being passed, hence its presence on the surface only. Bleeding into the rectum gives time for some mixing of blood and faeces before its expulsion. James had noticed the bleeding was worse than before – a sign of an increase in growth of a possible tumour, rather than piles, bleeding from which is likely to stay at a similar level.

As for his weight, he wasn't in the habit of weighing himself, so he didn't know if it had changed. He had noticed, however, that his trousers were a bit looser on him. He had had to take his belt in a notch or two recently. His wife thought he was a bit thinner in the face. And he was more tired than he used to be after finishing a shift in the brewery. He put that down to his advancing age. His work involved dealing with heavy barrels and shovelling malt, so it was very physical.

So far, the answers he had given were not what I wanted to hear. I asked him if he had any other problems he would like to discuss. He actually laughed, and asked me if I thought the probable diagnosis of cancer wasn't enough for one person. I agreed that it was, but he accepted that I had to question him a little further, even if it were just to practise what I had been learning about taking a full history from patients.

No, he hadn't had any other serious illnesses or operations. He had never been a patient in a hospital before, in his whole life. Yes, he smoked around 30 cigarettes a day and drank a few beers most evenings. He worked in a brewery, and in those days the workers were given a few free beers every day. He (and all his workmates) took advantage of his employers' generosity. As for his family, his father had died in his fifties of a heart attack, and his mother had had to have her bowel removed, he had been told, 'for an ulcer'. She had died, aged 47, two years later 'from complications of her operation'. No one in the family knew what kind of ulcer it was, but she had had a colostomy. James had no brothers or sisters.

I took note of all these answers, but it was many years before I understood their significance. At that time, as I have already explained, they were just the routine questions we medical students had been trained to ask of every patient, not just those with possible cancer. The routine goes like this:

PCO – 'Patient Complaining Of'. This is the symptom or symptoms that have brought the patient to the doctor. In James's case, the main symptom was rectal bleeding.

HPC – 'History of Present Complaint'. This is how long the symptoms have been present, how they have varied in that time, and what the patient has tried to do about them (or not, as was often the case in those days).

PMH – 'Personal Medical History'. This is the patient's past illnesses, and how they may or may not relate to the current problem. It includes smoking and drinking habits and other aspects of lifestyle, such as exercise and drug taking. James was not taking any prescribed drugs for any chronic illness, nor was he ever inclined to buy pills for various aches and pains 'over the counter'. He had not had any reason to do so.

PSH – 'Past Surgical History'. This is an account of the patient's previous operations – from removal of tonsils or appendix as a child, to operations needed as an adult for illnesses or accidents.

FH – 'Family History'. This encompasses the medical problems and illnesses of the patient's immediate family – parents, grandparents, uncles, aunts, siblings and children. They may well give a clue to the current illness.

SH – 'Social History'. This includes the patient's occupation, and an assessment of the area in which he or she lives. In the past it was usual to define patients by their social class. Political correctness today makes that less easy, and less emphasis is put upon it as the class divisions have blurred over the years.

Having completed all these sections of the history-taking, I then had to examine the patient. Strictly, at this stage we were not supposed to come to any conclusions about the possible diagnosis, but that's hard to avoid in a case like James's. The history alone was enough to make the diagnosis of cancer probable. Here was a man who had never had a previous illness who was suddenly passing blood with his stools. The best we could hope for was that he had grown a polyp or two in the bowel, that had not yet turned malignant. He was already too old for the start of ulcerative diseases of the bowel such as ulcerative colitis, most cases of which begin in the teens or early adulthood. We already knew from his GP that haemorrhoids (piles) were not the cause.

Faced with the passage of blood per rectum by an older man with no previous history of bowel illnesses, doctors must put bowel cancer at the top of the list of suspect diagnoses. What we didn't know then, but most certainly do know now, is that there were several more pointers to probable bowel cancer in James's history. He was a smoker – tobacco is a powerful inducer of cancer, just as much of the bowel as of the lung. He drank fairly heavily, even though he was rarely drunk. Heavy drinking, too, is a bowel cancer promoter. His lack of previous history of bowel disease was also a pointer: it virtually ruled out one of the common inflammatory bowel diseases, such as Crohn's or ulcerative colitis. As he hadn't taken any patent medicines or prescription drugs, we could rule out bleeding from a drug reaction.

His family history gave a clue, too. Just why did his mother have her colon removed? Was the 'ulcer' really a bowel cancer? It was common in those days for doctors to keep the diagnosis of cancer a secret from people, because it was thought unkind to label them with what was then considered to be a lethal disease. So the euphemism 'ulcer' was used instead, even to the rest of the family. On the other hand, his mother might have had bleeding polyps, for which total colectomy might have been essential to save her life. She might have had familial adenomatous polyposis (FAP). If so, James could have inherited it from her, and also have inherited its potential to turn malignant.

James obviously needed a thorough examination, first of his abdomen, then his rectum. His abdomen was flat; he was slim, despite his prodigious alcohol consumption – another pointer, perhaps, to cancer. He might well have lost weight without knowing it. There were no abnormal lumps to feel – always a good sign – but he was tender when I pressed on the lower left quarter of his abdomen, below and to the left of the navel. That part of his abdomen felt just a little more resistant to pressure over it than the corresponding opposite side. This is quite common in someone who is constipated – mostly the resistance is just a firm stool awaiting expulsion at the next visit to the toilet. But the tenderness was ominous.

Rectal examination added to my disquiet. Instead of the usual soft lining of the rectum I could feel on one side of it a hard thickened area. That, too, was uncomfortable for him, but not actually painful. When I withdrew my finger, there was a smear of blood on the tip of the glove.

The Professor came round the screen at that moment, and called me away. In those days, there was no talking in front of the patient. He asked me what I had found, and I had to say I thought he had a cancer of the rectum, that had formed a half-circle around it, and was beginning to narrow the bowel lumen. He agreed, and asked me to wait and hear what he had to say to James.

In those days there were no flexible endoscopes and diagnoses were made by simple examination. The tumour, if it was low enough in the colon, might have been seen with the use of a rigid endoscope, but if it was further up (beyond the sigmoid) it could only be viewed and assessed indirectly by using a barium enema. James's only hope was to be treated by a surgeon who knew how to interpret the physical signs and X-rays accurately, could remove the tumour completely and safely, and would hope that it had not spread beyond the bowel wall into the abdominal cavity and perhaps further, into the liver and other organs. There was no ultrasound assessment of the tumour spread, and no blood tests whereby we could measure the extent of the cancer.

So James was told that he would be put on the surgical list in two days' time – enough to 'clean' the bowel so that the operation would not put him at risk of infection afterwards. Then, too, we did not have the wide range of antibiotics with which to treat possible infections after surgery. The Professor also told him, as was the practice at the time, that he had some 'trouble' in the bowel that had to be removed, or it might become 'nasty' in the future. The words 'cancer' and 'tumour' were not mentioned. They were considered too frightening for the patient to comprehend or to live with. The fact that James had used the word to me did not seem to matter to the Professor. In retrospect, I believe that the avoidance of the truth and its unpleasant implications was really to protect the Professor himself, rather than the patient, from having to go through with a very difficult discussion.

James turned out to be one of the lucky ones, in that he survived. His operation was a success. He was given a colostomy and, despite the relatively long history of symptoms, he left hospital with no obvious remnant of cancer in his bowel or abdomen. I saw him at the follow-up clinic two years later, and he was still well. For that time, this was a very good result.

Over the years since then, the history-taking has not changed, nor has the initial physical examination. The *big* advances have been made in the further tests made to confirm the diagnosis and to assess the nature of the tumour we find. By the time we treat colorectal cancers we know its type, its size, its spread and how best we can manage it, from surgery to chemotherapy and beyond. Most of all, we talk honestly and openly with our patients, in a partnership against the illness. This makes for a more trusting and closer relationship between patient and doctor that carries on through all the possible complications and setbacks of the fight against the disease.

It is so much easier to tell the truth, rather than try to remember to repeat the lies that have to be told again and again at each subsequent consultation between doctor and patient.

Two 'near misses'

Even with all this knowledge, we can still miss a diagnosis. I remember two women in their sixties, who presented in the same way more than 30 years apart. Their diagnosis was missed for several months, and the delay must have materially altered their chances of surviving.

Mary

Mary was a farmer's wife. Her husband had had to retire early (for a farmer) three years before, after a stroke had left him partially paralysed and with difficulty talking and feeding himself. Mary had taken on the role of carer, helping him rise every morning, feeding him, washing him, and generally caring for him until night-time. Naturally, the extra physical work and mental anguish took their toll. She had lost 13 kilos (about 2 stone) in weight, and felt tired all the time. Her sister, a retired nurse, told her that she was just doing too much, and that the tiredness and weight loss were simply the result of her physical burden and her advancing age.

So when it was eventually arranged for Mr Duncan to go into a care home for two weeks, to give the two sisters a holiday, nothing was said to me, Mary's doctor, about her weight loss and fatigue. The doctor in charge of the admission to the care home didn't know Mary very well, because he was only her husband's doctor, not hers. That was a relic of country practice in those days – when people got married they tended to stick to their old doctors. And as the doctors were often in competition for patients, they tended not to share information. So Mr Duncan's doctor didn't know about Mary's malaise, and I hadn't been told about her husband's illness. I had actually never met Mary, because I had only moved into the practice a year before, and she had never had occasion to visit me.

Mary then went on holiday without my knowing anything about her problems. It was only afterwards, when her sister realized that Mary's health wasn't 'picking up' during the holiday, that she suggested she see her doctor. It took another week or so before Mary agreed.

In Mary's case, the presenting symptom (PCO – remember the routine from page 38?) had nothing to do with the bowel. She just felt tired all the time, and was feeling generally unwell. She couldn't put her finger on what was wrong, but she agreed that she had been 'overdoing it' for many months. She had little time to herself, and spent all her waking hours tending to her husband. Wasn't she entitled, she asked me, to feel a little down?

Having heard of the magnitude of her problems at home, I was inclined to agree with this. But I asked the usual questions anyway. How long had she been feeling like this? For around three months. Had she had any other symptoms that seemed relevant? Only that she had lost her appetite and consequently was eating less – perhaps that had caused her to lose weight. She had no aches and pains, and opening her bowels and passing urine were just as they had always been.

Mary had always been healthy, didn't smoke or drink, and her only previous admissions to hospital had been for the births of her babies. She had always been on the heavy side, and she blamed that on the fact that her farmer husband had always needed a lot of food and 'had a healthy appetite'. She had eaten the same amount as him all their married life – and this meant a hearty breakfast, a 'good lunch' and a 'proper evening meal'. In between there was plenty of farmhouse baking, with scones, cakes and biscuits on the table whenever they were wanted by the 'menfolk'. This last word was hers, not mine – and was a normal attitude in farming households in those days. So, not unnaturally, the womenfolk ate their fair share. Their two daughters and one son were all on the heavy side, thanks to their upbringing.

Her mother was still alive in her nineties, in a care home, but apparently well. Mary's father had died of a heart attack in his seventies.

My first thought was that Mary's symptoms were all about her workload, and perhaps depression too. Indeed, all her symptoms could easily have been attributed to depression, and there was no pointer to any physical illness. However, she was pale and drawn, even verging on the thin side. Having never seen Mary before, I couldn't help feeling that this was not the appearance of a farmer's wife who had eaten well all her life. Depression alone would have been unlikely to have wrought such a radical change.

A full physical examination revealed little. Her heart and lungs were normal, as was her blood pressure. Her abdomen was soft with no obvious masses or tenderness, and she had no problems in her nervous system. The probable diagnosis from these findings was still depression and exhaustion, but I wasn't completely convinced. A simple urine test to look for glucose (to rule out diabetes) and albumin (to exclude kidney disease) was negative. There was no blood in the urine, nor were there any signs of infection. Urinary infection is often a cause of malaise in older women, and that too was one of the diagnoses to be ruled out. So to make absolutely certain that I wasn't missing something, I took a blood test, to check whether or not she was anaemic – anaemia being another possible cause for her symptoms. She was asked to come back in two days for the results.

I wasn't really surprised when I saw them – she had severe anaemia. Her haemoglobin level, which is a measure of the red pigment in the red blood cells that carry oxygen around the body, was only 8 grams per decilitre. This was only just over half what it should have been. The cells were smaller than normal, and the microscope slide showed a few immature red cells, or *reticulocytes*, in the blood picture. This is a sign that the bone marrow is working harder than normal to replace blood that is being lost.

I had to question Mary again, this time directly about possible causes of the blood loss. She had not been bleeding as far as she knew. Her stools were the normal colour and the usual consistency. She had been a bit breathless going upstairs, but she thought that was 'just her age'. She couldn't remember the last time she had to run for anything, so she didn't know if she was breathless on exertion.

Anaemia is not a diagnosis in itself – it is a pointer to an illness. If you are anaemic, you are either not digesting enough iron and proteins to make enough haemoglobin, or your bone marrow, for some reason, is not making enough because it is abnormal, or you are losing blood faster than you can make it. That seemed to be the case for Mary. So from where was she losing the blood?

The most likely place was in the stool. If we are losing a small amount of blood every day, say a teaspoonful, from our bowel, it may well not be noticed. Yet if we do that over many months we will become anaemic. There are tests that can be applied to the stool that will detect this 'occult' (i.e. hidden) bleeding – and that was the next step for Mary. She was asked to take three small pots home with her, and instructed how to place a small amount of stool, using a special spatula, into the pot on successive days. The test results would quickly show if she was losing blood.

Each test did prove positive for occult blood, so her case had now become urgent. We had to assume that she had something in her large bowel that was causing her to bleed and, at her age and under such stress, it had also to be assumed that it was likely to be malignant.

Mary was referred urgently to the local gastro-enterology team, who found from barium studies that she had a large cancer in her caecum, the first part of the colon, in the right lower quarter of her abdomen. Today she would have had an ultrasound test that would have saved her from having to have a bowel filled with barium, but this development was still 20 years ahead of us then.

Sadly, on opening her abdomen at the operation, the tumour was seen to have spread to the under surface of her liver. At that time, too, nothing could be done after a tumour had spread beyond the site at which it had grown. No attempt was made to remove the cancer, and she was 'closed up' in the theatre. Mary lived only a month after her operation.

Jane

Mary's cancer occurred in the early 1970s. Thirty years later, I had to deal with Jane. A schoolteacher, she had led an active life until after she retired at 60. She was only one year into her retirement when her husband, John, who was nine years her senior, was given the diagnosis of Alzheimer's disease. Like Mary, 30 years before, all Jane's energies went into looking after her husband. The Alzheimer's Society helped to provide carers to let her get away for a few hours every day, so that she could spend some time with friends, her son and her grandchildren. It was the family who brought her to my notice.

They were worried that she was getting thinner and complaining of stomach pains that she had assumed were caused by 'indigestion'. They were concerned that she was getting through packs of over-the-counter antacids every week, but they were not helping much. She had also stopped smoking – something, like many teachers, she had failed to do when still at work. Yet she was reluctant to see me, because she assumed, just like Mary had 30 years before, that her tiredness and feeling ill were merely the result of having to care for her husband.

One look at Jane was enough to worry me. She had certainly lost weight since the last time I had seen her, which was only a month before, in a routine meeting to discuss her husband's care. Like Mary, she had lost her appetite. But, unlike Mary, she had some abdominal symptoms. She was tender over the left side of her abdomen, to the side and just below the navel. There was a fullness there that wasn't present on the right side. More ominously, she was also tender in the upper right side of her abdomen, just under the right rib margin. This is usually a sign of liver or gallbladder problems.

Jane then admitted to me that she hadn't felt well for at least six months, and had actually lost more than 20 kilos (around 3 stone) in weight over the last three months. She had not noticed any change in her bowel movements, or bleeding, nor had her urine flow altered. Asked why she had stopped smoking, she said she had 'lost her taste for them'. She had never had any bowel problem before. Her only past medical history was of fairly severe asthma in her middle age that had necessitated her taking steroid pills for several months each year. However, she had had no attacks, and no treatment for her asthma, for around ten years.

Rectal examination was difficult to assess. I wasn't sure whether or not I could feel something just within reach of my finger, in the last part of the colon. In our region of Scotland, we can order an urgent ultrasound examination direct from practice in our local hospital. This was arranged for two days' time, and a stool sample was sent to the lab.

The results were not good. The stool did contain blood, and the ultrasound showed a mass in the descending colon, just where I thought I could feel it. Worse, the tender area under the right ribs showed a problem, probably another mass, in the lower margin of the liver. I was reminded of Mary, 30 years before.

However, 30 years is a long time in medicine. Jane was admitted and investigated further. The 'spot' in the liver seemed to be a solitary secondary tumour, and at operation she had both the primary and secondary tumours removed. She was given a colostomy, and then offered chemotherapy to 'hit' any residual cancer.

She thought about refusing it, as she knew very well that the chemotherapy would not be pleasant. But she decided to accept it, because it would give her more than an even chance of continuing to look after John.

It is now a year since Jane finished her chemotherapy, and she is almost back to her old self, and still looking after John. We don't know how long we can keep any residual cancer cells at bay, but do know that if it recurs we have something in hand to offer as treatment. She remains optimistic that she has beaten the disease. We are not so sure, but at least she has had more quality time than we were able to offer Mary, three decades ago.

Looking back at Jane's case, we may wonder why she should have developed bowel cancer. Did it have anything to do with her smoking? Had the stresses inherent in looking after a much-loved husband with Alzheimer's disease something to do with it? Was there an inherited aspect to the initiation of her illness? That was difficult to assess, because her father had been killed in the Second World War, and her mother had died of old age in her ninety-ninth year. What Jane ate may have had something to do with it. She always admitted that she was the 'world's worst cook' and had bought in ready-cooked meals for her family. She had found as a teacher that spending time cooking complicated meals was a distraction she could do without as she had to mark pupils' work in the evenings. For years, the family had been treated to the super-market's convenience foods and the wonders of the microwave. There is no way of knowing how what she ate affected her risk of bowel cancer, except to state that she had not had her fair share of fresh vegetables and fruits for many years.

After colitis

Lawrence

At 22, Lawrence Brown suddenly became very ill with severe diarrhoea, in which there was very heavy bleeding and copious amounts of mucus. It quickly became very obvious that he had ulcerative colitis, and that the only way to save his life was to remove his colon. His surgeons left in a 'stump' of rectum and anus, in the hope that one day they would be able to link it up again with his ileum, so that he could have a functioning anus.

Lawrence improved greatly after his operation and learned to use his ileostomy so well that no one would have guessed that he had it. Yet he yearned, naturally, to be rid of it, and open his bowels naturally again. The rectal stump remained healthy, and eventually the surgeons linked up the two ends of bowel. For several years Lawrence was fine, with no troubles, except for the occasional bloody discharge from the anus on defaecation. He was followed up every year at the surgical clinic.

About ten years after the re-operation, however, the rectal wall began to look suspicious to the endoscopist. A biopsy of the site was taken, and it proved to be undergoing malignant change. The only answer was to remove it and to re-establish the ileostomy. Lawrence had to accept the decision, or face a very high risk of developing cancer in the stump.

To give him credit, he took the news very well. He had had an ileostomy before, and knew what was ahead of him. And he had half-expected the change, knowing from all he had read that ulcerative colitis is a pre-malignant condition. He is 49 now, and still well. He keeps fit in the gym, and still no one would know that he has an ileostomy.

Finding a lump

Walter

Walter was a successful business executive who was too busy to be ill. At 45, he was going places, travelling round the world, eating when he could, often on the hoof. His usual fare was made up of airline food, snatched breakfasts in hotels, and business dinners in restaurants. They were never regular and often eaten in time zones very different from his home.

He thought himself immune to illness, until he was asked by his company to undergo an insurance medical. The doctor doing it stopped when he felt Walter's abdomen. There was a firm lump below and to the right of his navel, that was not tender, and that Walter had never noticed. Yet it was around 5 centimetres (about 2 inches) in diameter – something you would have expected him to have felt in the normal course of living, even soaping himself in the bath.

But Walter was too busy to take baths – he had showers instead, and he spent as little time as possible in them. Sure enough, standing up, the lump was less easy to feel: it fell into the pelvis, so that it was understandable that it could have been missed.

To enter a room expecting to have a routine medical examination and to leave it with an urgent appointment for a specialist in bowel cancer is a shock to anyone, and Walter was probably more vulnerable than most. He had too much to do, he said, to take time off at the moment for investigations. Could it not wait until after the summer round of sales conferences?

He was gently told that if he waited, they might be his last conferences. The insurance doctor got his permission to phone his doctor, and the next week an ultrasound test confirmed a large tumour in the caecum. He had surgery the week after that. That was 15 years ago. It changed Walter's life. The realization that he was not pausing to 'smell the roses' made him think. He gave up his high-powered job and moved to a cottage in the country. The funds he made from selling his town house more than cushioned him from his loss of salary. He now tends his garden and, for a small fee, gardens for other people in his village. He doesn't miss his old lifestyle, and says he is happy. He is also an enthusiastic supporter of Cancer Research UK (CRUK), for which he uses his old marketing skills in rustling up funds.

Cramps – blocking the bowel

Rachel

Very occasionally, people ignore their symptoms until they develop into a full-scale emergency – and Rachel was an example of this. A very private lady, she had been a widow for many years. She had always had difficulties with her 'bowels', and had been in the habit of taking a laxative (she rang the changes between salts, syrup of figs and senna) every day since childhood. Her parents had been of the opinion that a daily 'clear out' was the best thing for a healthy life. Rachel saw no reason to change the habit, so was used to having 'stomach cramps' before opening her bowels. Indeed, she didn't feel as if she had had a complete day without some discomfort.

So when Rachel had a day when the cramps were really bad, she didn't think it too strange at first. Only when she realized that they were persisting much longer than usual, and that she could not empty her bowel, no matter how hard she tried, did she begin to panic. That evening she began to feel sick and very ill, and knew that she could not face the night without seeking medical help. The new NHS 24 service was in place, so her call was 'triaged' by a stranger on the phone, who quickly recognized that she needed urgent attention. An ambulance was called for her, and she was brought into the emergency call centre. There it was quickly realized that she had a complete colon obstruction. She had a tumour that had encircled her descending colon (on the left side of her abdomen), and the faeces had built up behind it. The pains were the result of her colon trying with no success to push its contents beyond the obstruction.

Rachel needed emergency surgery to relieve the obstruction. She was given a temporary colostomy with the intention of closing it off later, when the wound had healed. She had a difficult few days after the operation, but has recovered well in the longer term. It is unusual today for people to let things go so far that the cancer completely blocks the colon. But Rachel is a very private person, and tends to keep her symptoms to herself. That's a pity, because if she had come to the doctor earlier with her symptoms, she would have had a more comfortable time. It turned out that she had had more severe constipation than usual for around eight months before the episode that had brought her into hospital. She had just assumed, like many others do, that it was her age that had brought about the change in her bowel habit. Yet there is no 'normal' pattern of changing bowel habits as we grow older. If they change, we need to talk to a medical person about it. Age is not the sole cause – *ever.*

A changed bowel habit

Polly

A few weeks after the experience with Rachel, Polly appeared at our 'Well Woman Clinic'. The practice nurse performs a smear and checks the breasts and blood pressure, tests the urine for diabetes and kidney disease, and asks about any relevant symptoms. Polly looked the picture of health, and it was only as she was leaving the room she turned back and said that she had had one small problem. For the last two months she had been constipated for the first time in her life. Instead of 'going' every day after breakfast, her frequency was down to once or twice a week. Her stools had become very hard and difficult to pass.

The nurse called me in, and we went over in detail what other changes in Polly's lifestyle might have caused this change. It seemed that there were none. There was nothing for it but to examine her. Just at the colorectal junction I could feel a firm ring of what felt like hard muscle completely encircling the bowel. I hoped that this was not a repeat of Rachel's problem, and phoned our local consultant's secretary. She was given an endoscopy appointment in three days' time.

Naturally Polly was concerned that I had arranged an endoscopy so quickly. I was obviously taking her symptoms more seriously than she had thought they merited. I explained that I thought that she had a spasm of the muscles of the rectum, but that I could not rule out something 'more serious'. She knew what that meant.

Polly spent three anxious days before her endoscopy. Happily, the consultant confirmed that she did have an extreme form of irritable bowel, and that the constipation was nothing more than spasm of muscles in a normal bowel. Not all that seems to be malignant turns out to be so bad, and irritable bowel is a much more common finding in gastro-enterological clinics than cancer.

The clotting veins

Alan

Alan was 59 when he first noticed a health problem. It wasn't to do with his bowel, but his legs. A day after arriving home from a business trip to the west coast of the United States, he noticed that his left leg was swollen and tender below the knee. It was clearly a deep vein thrombosis in the calf, for which he had to be given warfarin treatment. This surprised him, as he had taken all the usual advice about flying long distances, including wearing support stockings, drinking plenty of water beforehand and on the flight, and avoiding alcohol. He also travelled business class, so had been able to stretch out on the night flight eastwards across North America and the Atlantic.

Nevertheless, the thrombosis was blamed on the long flight and he was given first an intravenous infusion to disperse the clot and then put on a low dose of warfarin for a few weeks until the swelling disappeared. He was asked to stop smoking, a powerful promoter of deep vein thrombosis, but he found this difficult to do. He had been a smoker since his mid-teens, and because he had been healthy until now he had never seen the need to stop. He assumed that the bad effects of smoking 'would never happen to him'.

For about three weeks, Alan did well. His leg felt better, and he returned to work in his office. Then he noticed a swelling in his right calf. This time there had been no long flight beforehand, and it alarmed him. His doctor confirmed that he had another thrombosis. Repeated thromboses in a person with no known cause has to be regarded as suspicious, as they can be a sign of a hidden cancer. Usually it is in the lung, but colorectal cancer can also be linked to them.

Because of his smoking history, his GP asked for a chest X-ray and ordered a full blood count. With a haemoglobin of 11.8 G/dl he was moderately anaemic for a previously healthy male. That raised his doctor's suspicions further and he was asked to give three faecal specimens for occult blood. Each one of them showed positive.

Alan had had no symptoms at all that could be linked to his bowel, yet an ultrasound examination showed he had a tumour in his caecum. Happily, it could be removed entirely, and at operation there was no sign of spread either locally into the peritoneum or to the liver or other organs in his abdomen. After recovery from the operation, there were no further clotting incidents. He has not smoked since.

At the time of writing this, three months after his operation, Alan is doing well. He has changed his job, doesn't commute or travel any longer, and has a very different outlook on life. As he says, 'The experience has stopped me chasing that elusive pot of gold. I want to enjoy life while I can.' He has a good chance of doing so for many years yet.

These case histories are all from my own experience, but any doctor would be able to add many more. They are included here to demonstrate the variety of ways in which colorectal cancer can arise, and also to show that the diagnosis need not be a death sentence. It is important, however, to have a 'low threshold of suspicion' if anything goes wrong with your gut. If you are experiencing anything like the symptoms described in the above case histories, please see your doctor.

7

How doctors diagnose bowel cancer

Reading the previous chapter you could be forgiven for thinking that bowel cancer can arise in so many ways, and that it is mimicked by so many other problems, that it is either very difficult to spot, or that it is suspected in virtually every patient who goes to their doctor! This recognition that it can present in so many forms has led doctors to follow quite strict guidelines in making the diagnosis. They are summarized in this chapter.

Symptoms

First, people may have so few symptoms early on in the disease that the cancer can grow for a long time before spreading beyond the inner lining of the bowel. It is true that younger patients are more likely than older ones to notice symptoms, but they are likely to delay going to their doctor because they think they can't be indicative of a serious illness. Older people may be slower to notice their symptoms, but when they do, they go to their doctors earlier. So it is important for anyone, young or old, to realize that any new symptoms related to the bowel or to their general well-being should be reported to their doctor as soon as possible.

Often the symptoms will not carry such a serious outlook. As an example of this, the classical illness that brings most people with abdominal symptoms to their doctor is irritable bowel syndrome (IBS). Because it is often difficult to persuade people with IBS that they don't have cancer, I have devoted the next chapter to it.

The main symptoms of bowel cancer in people over 45 are listed here.

- Change of the regular bowel habit to passing stools, usually loose, more often each day, for six weeks. (Diarrhoea that lasts for a shorter time is usually either an infection or a bout of irritable bowel.)
- Bleeding from the back passage without symptoms related to the anus, such as itching, soreness, discomfort, lumps (usually haemorrhoids or piles) and pain.

53

- Pain in the abdomen that persists all the time and does not respond to any painkillers or antacids.
- 'Tenesmus' – a strong, urgent desire to defaecate, but without being able to pass a motion. This may be a sign of a tumour low in the rectum.
- Faecal incontinence – the involuntary leaking of faeces from the anus.
- Unexplained anaemia, with or without any or all of these symptoms.

Doctors faced with patients with a combination of two or more of these symptoms will feel the abdomen and perform a rectal examination. They may feel a mass in the lower abdomen, on either side, or in the rectum itself. However, the examination may reveal no abnormal masses. That does *not* preclude sending the patient for tests. If there is any suspicion of bowel cancer in the doctor's mind, then it is imperative that the patient is seen in a specialist unit.

Referral

The list given above seems clear. However, the problem with it is that many people discover that they are bleeding from the anus, have noticed changes in their bowel habit and have regular pain in the abdomen, yet only a few of them are actually found to have colorectal cancer. In August 2003, Dr M. R. Thompson and his colleagues of the Queen Alexandra Hospital, Portsmouth, reviewed the extent and causes of bowel symptoms in people in the community and in hospital outpatients clinics (Thompson and colleagues, 2003, pp. 263–5). They found that more than 80 per cent of people with pain, bleeding and bowel habit changes do not see their doctors, and that these symptoms disappear without treatment.

Of those who do bother to visit their GP, under half are referred to hospital. They calculated that of people with rectal bleeding who don't see their doctor, the risk of cancer is 1 in 700. The risk rises to 1 in 30 among those who come to their doctor, and is 1 in 16 for people with bleeding who are referred to hospital surgical clinics. This last figure may seem high, but it means, of course, that 15 of every 16 referred to a clinic because cancer is suspected do not have the disease, and that 97 per cent of people seen with rectal bleeding in the GP's surgery do *not* have cancer. Put another way, only 3 in every 100 *do* have cancer. Most of the others have haemorrhoids.

Dr Thompson's team reasoned, justifiably, that so many ultimately unnecessary referrals to hospital delay the efficient investigation of people who actually have cancer, delay the reassurance of people without cancer, and block resources for the higher-risk patients. These referrals take up much needed medical and nursing time, and the patients themselves have to take time off work to be investigated, most of them unnecessarily. These disadvantages have, of course, to be weighed against the early diagnosis of the 1 in 16 patients who does have cancer.

Dr Thompson and his team therefore laid down seven key principles of 'watchful waiting' for people with bowel symptoms. These principles require the doctor to:

- establish the degree of concern and estimate the cancer risk from the patient's history and examination;
- adjust the period of watchful waiting to the patient's risk (for example, a patient who has had bleeding for six weeks should be fast-tracked to a surgical clinic; one with lower-risk symptoms can wait longer);
- ensure the patient understands the benefits of not being immediately referred;
- recognize the importance of the way the information is framed and emphasize it in writing;
- use a diagnostic test (such as faecal blood tests) if there is any doubt about the diagnosis and repeat the history and examination at frequent intervals while waiting for the clinic appointment;
- refer lower-risk patients who do not want to watch and wait to a routine clinic with an urgent appointment;
- ultimately refer all patients with persistent symptoms.

Dr Thompson and his colleagues agree that it is important for the public to be made aware of the risks of colorectal cancer, but they also point out that even a small increase in the number of patients presenting to general practice as a result of campaigns can have a large effect on the demand for hospital resources. Such campaigns, they argue, may even 'cause considerable harm in vulnerable patients without cancer by labelling them as being at risk. They need to make it clear that initial treatment with the help of a pharmacist is appropriate and may avoid unnecessary and occasionally harmful investigation.' They continue: 'In attempting to achieve prompt diagnosis of bowel cancer, doctors should not forget their responsibility to protect the much larger group of patients with benign disease from unnecessary investigation and from overburdening an already overstretched secondary care (i.e. hospital) system.'

Tests and examinations

When you do reach the clinic you will be offered a colonoscopy. You take a strong laxative the previous evening, and are examined the next day, when the bowel is empty and the bowel wall can be clearly seen. A flexible fibre-optic endoscope is used. It is not painful and, if you wish, you can even watch the progress of the examination inside your bowel on a television screen while it happens. There is usually no need to be sedated or tranquillized beforehand.

Colonoscopy is a very sensitive test. Studies have established that it will identify 96.7 per cent of cancers, 85.0 per cent of large polyps, and 78.5 per cent of small polyps. It does have some disadvantages, in that endoscopists are unable to see as far round the colon as the caecum in up to 30 per cent of patients. There are a very few cancers that can't be seen using the endoscope, and it may be difficult to tell exactly where in the bowel a tumour is.

To be sure of the diagnosis, a small piece, a 'biopsy', is removed from a possible tumour to examine microscopically, and perhaps to culture cells. Very occasionally this can lead to complications such as a hole in the bowel (a perforation). Overall, though, it remains a very safe investigation, with fewer than 1 in 17,000 colonoscopies leading to the death of the subject. Even that may sound a risk, but bear in mind that some colonoscopies are performed in seriously ill people with very fragile bowel walls.

Some patients are offered a double contrast barium enema, which is a bit less comfortable than a colonoscopy. Even so, there is no need for sedation. It is very safe, with a mortality of 1 in 57,000. However, its accuracy is reduced if patients have diverticular disease of the sigmoid colon, about which you will read in the chapter on irritable bowel.

A highly sensitive investigation is computed tomography pneumocolon, in which air is pumped into the colon and a 'CAT' scan used to scrutinize the bowel wall for polyps. It does not detect polyps under 10 millimetres in diameter, and is only available in specialist units where there is a fast computed tomography scanner. It is mostly reserved for people who are frail and less mobile than normal.

If a diagnosis of cancer is made, it is essential to define the limits of the disease. In Britain we use the Dukes' classification system, which asks four questions:

1 Is it confined to the lining of the gut at one site (the mucosa and submucosa, which is the layer of tissue just underneath the mucosa)? If so, this is Dukes stage A.
2 Has it eroded through the entire bowel wall? If so, this is Dukes stage B.
3 Has it spread to the local lymph glands next to the tumour? If so, it becomes Dukes stage C.
4 Has it spread beyond the lymph glands to distant organs, such as the liver? If so, it becomes Dukes stage D.

The stage of the tumour determines how it is to be treated. That is accomplished by computed tomography (CAT scan) or by magnetic resonance imaging (MRI scan). CAT scans are used chiefly to spot distant spread – as in Dukes' stage D. MRI scans are more useful in pinpointing local spread, particularly around the rectum and sigmoid area.

How colorectal cancer is treated is described in Chapter 9, but first we must get other diagnoses out of the way. The next chapter deals with those illnesses that are often mistaken for bowel cancer – irritable bowel and coeliac disease.

8

Irritable bowel, coeliac disease and diverticular disease

I pondered for a long time on whether to include a chapter on diseases other than colorectal cancer in this book. For those of you who *know* you have bowel cancer, it is probably an unnecessary section that may even annoy, because it seems so trivial in comparison with a malignancy. However, I decided to put it in because there are so many people who fear they have cancer, when in fact they have irritable bowel syndrome, adult coeliac disease or diverticular disease. They are so convinced that they have a lethal disease that it is often impossible to persuade them otherwise. So it is probable that many people who have one of these chronic bowel problems will buy this book, either to confirm to themselves that they have cancer or, hopefully, to be reassured that they have not.

Irritable bowel

I have had a long and not entirely successful relationship with irritable bowel. I was a student under Mr Brian Brooke, consultant surgeon at the Queen Elizabeth Hospital in Birmingham, and later Professor of Surgery at St George's Hospital in London. In his 1986 textbook, *The Troubled Gut*, he devotes only two pages to irritable bowel. He describes it as a 'strange equivocal condition seen all too often in gastrointestinal clinics throughout the world'. I remember Professor Brooke's frustration at the patients with irritable bowel who came to him believing they had something worse. He was often the second or third consultant they had visited, because they would not believe the opinions of lesser, more mortal, physicians. He saw irritable bowel sufferers as wasting his time, when he wanted to get on with treating people whom he saw as having 'real' problems – his cancer and colitis patients.

In a way, he was right. He writes that, 'The best treatment for irritable bowel lies with the doctor who is prepared to listen, who is able to recognize the condition from the story, who has the strength of mind to avoid recourse to investigation, and last but not least who will spend as much time as is needed to explain the situation. It is remarkable how the symptoms ease to tolerable proportions, if not totally, when suspicion and fear are properly allayed.' His clinic was not one in which the doctor could spend the time needed to help patients with irritable bowel.

My views on irritable bowel as a young GP were modelled on Professor Brooke's. Whenever people came to me with new symptoms that might be due to irritable bowel, I tried to take time to talk to them about the illness, and to avoid, whenever I could, sending them for investigations. That wasn't easy, because we had no clear, proven treatment for irritable bowel, and the patients naturally kept coming back. The fact that I could do little for them made them think the diagnosis was being missed. The result? In the end, most of them did make the journey up to hospital, to see our gastro-enterologists, who soon made the same diagnosis, and sent them back to me, no better, and little the wiser.

After six years in general practice, I decided to enter medical research. One of my first jobs was to help to develop the first drug specifically designed to help irritable bowel. This was mebeverine, otherwise known as Colofac.

It wasn't long before I came up against an almost insoluble problem. How could I measure the intensity of episodes of irritable bowel in such a way as to be able to analyse the results mathematically? We had to find a way of putting numbers on symptoms and signs, and then measuring the difference after treatment with the drug or placebo. Irritable bowel symptoms are not easily enumerated. The main ones are abdominal discomfort, bloating, and changes in the pattern and number of the bowel movements. The problem was that sometimes two different patients would describe the same type of bowel movement in two different ways. What would you call the passing of a shower of small hard pellets like rabbit droppings? We found some people called it constipation, while others were sure it was diarrhoea. As for putting numbers on discomfort in the abdomen, or the need to strain to pass a motion, our statistician would quietly sit in a corner and weep!

The 'fartometer'

I was fortunate in having Dr John Cumming, doctor to the students at Reading University, as a colleague. John, sadly, died too young, but one instrument he left to posterity was his 'fartometer'. This was a microphone that was fixed to a belt that was strapped round the patient's midriff. The patient wore it for 24 hours, and recorded the sounds made by his gut throughout that time. We were left with hours of tapes, recording gurgles, rumbles and other sounds less easy to describe in a respectable book!

The idea of the fartometer was brilliant. We thought at the time that the more active a bowel was, the louder and more frequent would be the sounds we collected. The less active the bowel, the quieter the abdomen. We were confident that differences in the sound, loudness, quality or frequency would in some way relate to the symptoms of irritable bowel, although at that time we didn't know whether irritable bowel was the result of an overactive or underactive bowel.

What we actually found was a complete surprise. The fartometer was used in hundreds of subjects, some with, and some without, irritable bowel. However, absolutely nothing we heard bore any relationship to the symptoms of the disease. If the sounds that emanate from the abdomen were any indication of the activity of the bowel, then the symptoms of irritable bowel did not correlate with them. Irritable bowel was not a result of either an underactive or an overactive bowel. The symptoms could occur when the bowel was quiet or extremely noisy. And we could find no general difference in the bowel sound pattern between irritable bowel sufferers and those who had never had symptoms of the illness.

Where did that leave us? In the first place, without results to publish – so you are reading the outcome of that research for the first time, in this book. But it meant that if we were to find what causes the symptoms of irritable bowel, we had to use more sophisticated and scientific systems to measure them. The next step was to use an electronic 'pill' that measured pressures around it, and sent the results out by radio signals. The subject of the research swallowed the pill, which could then be followed on its journey through the body, repeatedly measuring the pressures around it in the stomach, small intestine and colon. Finally it was excreted, picked up and washed (thoroughly!) and used again by the next patient. (Honestly, these people did give their fully informed consent to the studies!) Nowadays, the pills are only used once and discarded.

The pressure studies didn't help much either. There was no convincing link between pressure inside the bowel and symptoms of irritable colon – the irritable colon sufferers showed the same patterns, and the same timing of passage from mouth to anus, as the volunteers without symptoms. We still did not have the concrete measurements we needed to perform proper statistical analysis on the benefits and drawbacks of our proposed treatment.

Eventually we had to rely on asking patients to write down their impressions of the severity and timing of their symptoms, and try to analyse the differences between the days on drugs and on placebo. The results were still unsatisfactory, as it was very difficult for patients to make this assessment reliably from day to day.

ROME II definition of IBS

So why was this research so difficult, when the condition is so common in every developed country? International committees have struggled for years to find ways of diagnosing irritable bowel reliably, while ruling out more serious diseases like Crohn's and ulcerative colitis, cancer of the bowel and coeliac disease. In 1999, this came to fruition when a working party from Europe and North America designed the ROME II criteria for making the diagnosis of irritable bowel (Thompson and colleagues, 1999, pp. 1143–7). You will see that the symptoms of irritable bowel overlap, to some extent, with those of colorectal cancer.

ROME II defines irritable bowel as follows:

- The patient has had, for 12 weeks, that need not be consecutive, in the previous 12 months, abdominal discomfort or pain with two of the following three features:
  – relief on defaecation;
  – onset linked to a change in the frequency of stools;
  – onset linked with a change in the appearance of the stool.

- Symptoms that support the diagnosis include:
  – fewer than three motions per week;
  – more than three motions per day;
  – hard or lumpy stools;
  – loose or watery stools;
  – need to strain to open the bowel;
  – the feeling of urgency (to have to rush to get to the toilet) to open the bowel;

- the passing of mucus (white, phlegm-like material) during a bowel movement;
- a bloated, swollen, full-feeling abdomen.

- Symptoms against the diagnosis of irritable bowel, and which should mean further investigations include:
  - weight loss;
  - bleeding along with the diarrhoea;
  - diarrhoea at night that disturbs sleep;
  - anaemia.

Looking at these criteria for a diagnosis of irritable bowel, it is not surprising that British GPs have estimated that around 15 per cent of the population have it. What ROME II is describing is how the bowel reacts the next day to the previous heavy night out. And, for many others, these symptoms may just be the bowel 'complaining' at a diet of fast food, too much to eat, too little of which is fruit, vegetable and fibre.

If you recognize your symptoms in this list, then you almost certainly have irritable bowel, not cancer, and do not need further investigations. But you may need a lot of advice about what and how much you eat and drink, and how much you exercise. You may also need help on how to cope with stress, because anxiety and depression both seem to be linked to irritable bowel symptoms, perhaps by giving us a heightened awareness of our inner workings. When we worry or are under stress, we feel our heart beating faster, our mouth and throat becoming drier, and our neck muscles tensing. Becoming aware of our insides churning is part of the same mechanism.

Some investigators, indeed, believe that irritable bowel is merely the patient becoming aware of his or her insides. Once you do become aware of your bowel making noises, it can become difficult to ignore it. I'm not sure I buy that message in its entirety. There may be some truth in it, but there is also no doubt that irritable bowel is a physical entity, and that it can be helped by drugs, as well as lifestyle advice.

Treatment

The current drugs that are licensed for use in irritable bowel in Britain still include mebeverine, my drug project from so many years ago. I'm pleased about that because it means that the drug was of use, despite all our fruitless efforts to prove that it worked. It acts directly on the bowel wall muscle, relieving cramp. Similar direct-acting antispasmodics are alverine and colpermine, this last being peppermint oil. Antispasmodics are mainly prescribed for people whose symptoms are mainly of abdominal spasms, cramps and pain, or with frequent bouts of diarrhoea. Laxatives such as lactulose (that do not cause the muscle of the bowel wall to constrict) are usually the drug of first choice for people whose main symptom is constipation. It goes without saying, however, that everyone with irritable bowel should look at their lifestyle, and not just depend on a prescription.

If you have irritable bowel, what you eat matters. The trouble is that for different people it matters in different ways. Some people need more fruit and fibre and less meat and dairy products to feel better. Others feel worse when they fill their colon with such residue, and feel better on a lighter diet that gives them a smaller stool. You will not know which type you are until you try both. Then it is up to you to be disciplined enough to keep to the eating habit that suits you most.

Coeliac disease

The last paragraph about irritable bowel and eating habits is the perfect entry to the section on coeliac disease, because if there is one cause of diarrhoea that depends absolutely on what you eat – or, more specifically, what you *don't* eat – it is coeliac disease. That was proved beyond doubt in 1945, when the retreating Nazis decided to starve the Dutch by taking almost all of the food grown in the Netherlands back to Germany. The whole Dutch people suffered terribly, and many were starving when the war ended in May.

Yet one group of children did remarkably well. Without bread or food made from flour, they suddenly began to grow and feel much healthier. They were the children with an illness, the cause of which was unknown, but was named coeliac disease. Children affected by it failed to grow, were thin and listless, and had daily diarrhoea. The diarrhoea was full of fat and was very unpleasant for the children. Few of them grew to maturity, with most dying of malnutrition in their later childhood.

The doctors looking after them in 1945 were staggered by their seemingly miraculous recovery when deprived of bread. Luckily, they came to the right conclusion and continued the ban on bread and wheat flour even after the end of the war, when they were again in plentiful supply. Soon after that, it became clear that children with coeliac disease were reacting badly to gluten, an ingredient of wheat flour, and of some other cereals. The usual healthy columns and crypts of their small intestinal mucosa were replaced by a thin, flat layer of cells that were obviously unhealthy, and unable to digest food residues properly and efficiently. When all gluten was excluded from their food, the small bowel soon recovered and the columns and crypts returned. The mucosal cells looked normal and functioned perfectly and normal digestion resumed. Children whose previous outlook had been grim could now look forward to a healthy and long life, provided they stayed off gluten.

Today, doctors are fully aware that children who are not thriving should be tested for coeliac disease, and few children with diarrhoea escape the net. Happily, they don't need to undergo endoscopy to make the diagnosis. People with coeliac disease carry in their blood substances called endomysial antibodies, or EMA. These can be identified by a standard blood test. Once EMA has been found in your blood, you can start on your gluten-free future, and feel better after only a day or two. Children with coeliac disease, once they stop eating gluten, grow like mushrooms (which, of course, are gluten-free).

So why is coeliac disease featured in a book on cancer? In the last few years we have come to recognize that some adults with diarrhoea have a form of coeliac disease that did not affect them in childhood. Their symptoms could be confused with irritable bowel syndrome.

In November 2001, David Sanders and his colleagues of the Royal Hallamshire Hospital in Sheffield reported on blood antibody tests in 300 patients consecutively attending their university clinic with all the symptoms of irritable bowel according to the ROME II criteria (Sanders and colleagues, 2001, pp. 1504–8). They compared them with 300 similar 'control' subjects without irritable bowel symptoms. Fourteen of the 300 patients, and two of the 300 controls, turned out to have adult coeliac disease. Eleven of the patients and both of the controls were positive for EMA. The three patients who had negative EMA results had *antigliadin* antibodies, another test that helps to confirm coeliac disease.

Dr Sanders's group advised from these results that people thought to have irritable bowel syndrome should have at least one investigation – an EMA test to rule out coeliac disease. Antigliadin tests may also be useful. They added that trying to diagnose adult coeliac disease from the symptoms was not so helpful. They found coeliac disease in 2 out of 62 irritable bowel patients in whom constipation dominated, in 4 out of 84 with mainly diarrhoea, and in 8 out of 154 patients in whom diarrhoea and constipation alternated.

Their report started a debate among experts. One, Roland Valori of the Gloucestershire Hospital, wrote that he was screening for coeliac disease more and more patients with a wide range of odd bowel symptoms that do not fit neatly into the ROME II criteria. He added that 'very few of my patients with unexplained gastro-enterological symptoms fit neatly into the ROME II criteria'. For him, 'selecting patients for investigations for coeliac disease will continue to depend on subtle factors that are not so easily measured by a set of diagnostic factors'.

So what is the message from this chapter? It is that, in general, if you have repeated symptoms that fit with irritable bowel syndrome, then you don't need to be investigated for every possible eventuality. You can believe your doctor and consultant if they are happy that there is nothing more wrong with you than irritable bowel disease. However, it would be worth asking them if they have excluded adult coeliac disease. Blood tests to check on antigliadins (gliadin is a constituent of gluten) are one way – the EMA test mentioned above.

It is important that the diagnosis is either made or ruled out, because adult coeliac disease is just as eminently treated as the childhood form. It responds extremely well and fast to exclusion of gluten from your food. People with adult coeliac disease usually have symptoms that suggest that they are not fully digesting their food. They have diarrhoea, a bloated abdomen, yet lose weight and become anaemic and show signs of vitamin deficiency. These are all reversed by gluten exclusion.

However, we are increasingly recognizing that there is a less typical, or 'silent', form of adult coeliac disease. These sufferers may have no bowel problems, but instead complain of tiredness, and tests show they have anaemia, osteoporosis, difficulty in walking ('ataxia') or peripheral neuropathy. People with peripheral neurop-athy complain of numbness, pins and needles, and weakness in their limbs. They may also have problems in knowing where their feet are in space (loss of 'position sense') and may lose their sense of detection of heat and cold. Amazingly, all these symptoms, which are related to lack of digestion of vitamins, disappear by simply avoiding gluten.

The 14 patients described by Dr Sanders probably fell into a group of people midway between the 'typical' and 'silent' adult coeliacs. They had a few bowel symptoms, but not enough to classify them as 'typical', and too many to be 'silent' cases. Doctors like myself will have to look out for them in future among our mass of people diagnosed with irritable bowel. And people with irritable bowel should know about it themselves, so that they can ask the right questions. Let us hope they always get the correct answers.

Diverticular disease

Diverticula are small outpouchings from the colonic wall. The best way to describe them is like the 'bleb' in a bicycle tyre that occurs when a weakness in the outer tyre allows the inner tube to balloon through it. It is much the same mechanism, as the mucosa (the lining) bulges through a weakness in the muscle layer of the bowel wall at a point where a blood vessel enters it. Almost all of us develop diverticuli if we live long enough. Around two-thirds of 80-year-olds possess them, but most cause no symptoms. They can be solitary or run into the hundreds. They vary in size from 5 millimetres to 2 centimetres (just under 1 inch) in diameter.

Normally they are not a problem, but they can become infected, or cause a bowel obstruction, or even perforate (rupture). Problems with diverticuli have risen over the last half-century as our consumption of fibre has fallen: most experts believe the two are connected, and that the loss of bulk in the stools has led to pressure rising in the colon, with the consequent inflation of balloon-like diverticula.

If there are symptoms, they usually arise as pain, mainly in the lower left quarter of the abdomen. The pain is worsened by eating, and diminished by passing wind or opening the bowels. Bloating and constipation is common as the symptoms overlap with irritable bowel. There is generally no blood in the stool.

Diverticulitis is an infection of a diverticulum, caused by a small amount of hard faeces lying in the pouch. In diverticulitis the pain is much worse than normal, and a rectal examination is very tender, unlike that in cancer. There is a fever, and the patients often have hot and cold sweats. It is treated with antibiotics and a clear liquid diet. When the symptoms have settled, usually within two to three days, the diagnosis is made by careful colonoscopy. Recurrences are common, so the patient is warned to see the doctor early if the symptoms return, so that treatment can be started promptly.

Severe complications of diverticuli include obstruction, abscesses and bleeding, so that the symptoms can mimic cancer. In fact, diverticuli are the second most common cause of rectal bleeding after haemorrhoids in older British men and women. Even though the diagnosis seems clear, repeated bleeding in someone with diverticuli should be investigated to rule out a cancerous change. Some authors have suggested that there is a link between diverticuli and colorectal cancer, but there is no evidence that cancers arise more commonly in a diverticulum than in other areas of the colon. The link may be that both are more common in people who have eaten very low amounts of fibre (vegetables and fruit) throughout their lives.

9

Treating colorectal cancer
– aiming for cure

In the past, the words 'cancer' and 'cure' didn't go together, but much has changed. The emphasis has certainly shifted from palliative care to increasingly sophisticated surgery. In around two-thirds of people with colorectal cancer, surgery is effective, removing the cancer and giving a real chance of cure – or at least several years without recurrence of the cancer. This chapter looks at the types of surgery that may be appropriate in colorectal cancer, depending on its stage.

Surgery

Once the colonoscopy and biopsy have confirmed the cancer, barium enema may be used to confirm the site of the tumour before the operation and ultrasound can be used to gauge its size and whether there is local or distant spread. The type of surgery performed depends on where the cancer is, its size, and whether it can be completely removed.

In November 2003, Dr Paris Tekkis, of St Mark's Hospital, Harrow, working with Dr Michael Thompson's group from Portsmouth, reported on a British National Study of Surgery in Colorectal Cancer (Tekkis and colleagues, 2003, pp. 1196–9). It followed the results of surgery in 8,077 patients in 73 hospitals in Great Britain and Ireland over one year. All 11 geographical regions in the United Kingdom were involved.

Ten different operations were listed. Patients whose tumours could be completely removed underwent complete removal of their tumours from the right or left side of the colon and of the rectum. Those whose cancers had progressed beyond the bowel wall were given palliative operations to relieve their symptoms of obstruction. It is encouraging that the vast majority of the patients could be offered complete tumour removal.

The main aim of the study was to check on mortality within a month after the surgery, and to relate it to the conditions of the patients beforehand. Considering that many of the patients had been ill, old and frail, the numbers of deaths were low. The patients were classified according to their age, sex, their ability to withstand an anaesthetic (using a grading devised by the American Society of Anesthesiology, or ASA), their cancer site, the type of surgery, their urgency, their Dukes's stage, and whether the cancer was removed or bypassed.

The results were impressive. Considering the poor health and high operative risk in this group of ill people, there were very few deaths. A rising ASA grading (meaning their risk of reacting badly to anaesthesia), along with a higher Dukes's stage, older age, and operating under an emergency (because of an obstruction or a perforation), tended to raise the operative risk, but the overall mortality was only 7.5 per cent. With a low ASA and Dukes's stage, it was as low as 2 per cent.

Dr Tekkis reported that in younger patients with less advanced cancers, removal of the area of bowel containing the tumour and re-uniting the bowel was very effective and led to very few deaths. In older patients with advanced cancer, trying to remove the whole tumour was more risky than performing a bypass operation and preparing a stoma, and leaving the cancer in place. One successful operation in such patients was the placing of a 'stent' inside the affected part of the colon. This keeps the colon open and allows passage of intestinal contents through it, avoiding obstruction. Such surgery gives the patients a better chance of a post-operative period of survival with a good quality of life.

Stents

It's probably useful here to explain stents in more detail. They are used in patients who have an obstruction in the bowel due either to a ring-shaped cancer running round the circumference of the lumen, or to a cancer that has grown from one side large enough to block the flow of faeces through it. A stent is placed in the bowel during an endoscopy, without the need for surgery. Like a firm but flexible hollow tube, it is passed in its unexpanded state using an endoscope through and beyond the site of the cancer. The endoscopy tube is then withdrawn, allowing the stent to expand to fill the bowel, compressing the cancer away from the lumen. This allows the free flow of faeces to return and to be maintained.

Inserting a stent is a huge relief to someone with an obstruction. It is particularly good for someone who is frail and who might not tolerate surgery well. Before the use of stents, the only way to unblock a bowel obstruction for cancer was to open the abdomen under an anaesthetic and bring to the surface a loop of colon above the obstruction. A colostomy was formed, and the bowel emptied through it. This has two serious disadvantages. One, of course, is the stress and strain, both physical and mental, of the operation. The second is the fact that the patient now has to get used to a colostomy, which is often difficult for older people who remain ill with cancer.

Stents address both of these problems. The patient can still defaecate normally and the stress is no more than a colonoscopy, which is usually only a minor discomfort, and is much less likely to cause complications or illness.

S. Gumovsky-Reicher and colleagues of Torrance, California, reported in 2003 (Gumovsky-Reicher and colleagues, 2003, p. 16) that self-expandable metal stents are effective and safe in patients whose colorectal cancers are causing an intestinal blockage. Over the previous five years they had used them in 48 patients. Eighty per cent of their patients were able to start eating normal food again within 36 hours of their stent insertion. None had any serious complications such as perforation or bleeding, and there were no deaths. Of those who were not a complete success, most could be treated after a further endoscopy.

Laparoscopy ('keyhole' surgery)

The operations in the British National Study used conventional 'open' surgical techniques. At the same time, Hong Kong surgeon Ka Lau Leung and colleagues were running a trial comparing conventional surgery with laparoscopic (popularly known as *keyhole*) surgery in 403 patients with rectosigmoid cancers. They reported their work in the *Lancet* of 10 April 2004 (Leung and colleagues, 2004, pp. 1187–92).

They proved that the keyhole method was as effective and safe as the open surgery. The laparoscopic method took longer to complete and was more expensive, but the post-operative recovery was faster and more comfortable for the patients. There were similar numbers of post-operative complications (40 for the laparoscope and 45 for conventional) in the two groups. There were only 9 deaths among the 403 patients, again very creditable in such a seriously ill sample of people. Just as hopeful is the fact that the Hong Kong doctors are predicting that more than three-quarters of their patients (75.3 per cent of the keyhole group, and 78.3 per cent of the conventional group) will be disease-free five years after their surgery.

German surgeons have come to similar conclusions to the Hong Kong group. Dr H. Scheidbach and colleagues, of Magdeburg, have reviewed their laparoscopic surgery patients with colorectal cancer from the time they began using the technique in 1991. They found that it was just as effective and complete as open abdominal surgery, and that the long-term results were at least as good. However, even in 2003 (Scheidbach and colleagues, 2003, pp. 439–46), they were unable to give it complete approval as the treatment of choice until more very large trials comparing the two techniques have been performed.

My own feeling is that the choice is best left up to your surgeon. If the team is very well versed in the keyhole technique, then that's fine and just as good as open surgery. But don't especially seek out a 'keyhole' surgeon just because it is keyhole. It is more important to choose the right surgeon for you, regardless of the method.

And follow-up . . .

Follow-up after surgery is important. If you have had a curative operation for colorectal cancer, do return for your follow-up visits. They may well prolong your life. That is the message from Andrew Renehan and his colleagues from hospitals in Manchester and Nottingham, who have analysed different follow-up regimens for people after colorectal cancer surgery.

They make the strong point that around one-third of colorectal cancer patients develop recurrences. This, of course, means that two-thirds are cured, which I suppose is a more positive way to look at the figures. However, they are concerned that the one-third who have a recurrence have it detected as soon as possible and have the most effective treatment for it.

They showed that intensive follow-up improved mortality from all causes within the first five years after surgery, and was cost-effective. They also showed that when a recurrence happened, those in the intensive follow-up group were more likely to be able to have curative, rather than just palliative, treatment for it. Intensive follow-up screening for colorectal cancer was at least as effective in improving long-term survival as it is for breast cancer.

Intensive follow-up isn't easy, though. It involves patients and doctors in regular meetings, with time and costs spent in laboratory tests, regular endoscopies, new polyp removal, drugs and all the costs of a busy X-ray department. If there is a recurrence, there are obvious surgical and other treatment costs. Yet all this trouble is worth it in that it does prolong lives and gives people good-quality survival. So if you are contemplating surgery, do remember that it is only the beginning of your fight against cancer – and that we do seem to be winning the battles, one by one. Remember that figure quoted at the beginning of this book: deaths among men with bowel cancer have fallen by 27 per cent, and among women by 43 per cent. These figures are almost entirely due to better and earlier detection of the cancers in the first place, to more effective surgery, and then to better follow-up after surgery.

Of course, being told that you need regular follow-up visits to make sure that your cancer hasn't returned is frightening, as it's natural to think that a returning cancer is a death sentence. The same goes for being told that your cancer couldn't all be removed, and that the operation has been one to relieve an obstruction and to make you more comfortable, rather than to cure you. If you are on this particular treadmill, the next two chapters are for you. They offer hope and, with each year that passes, research teams all over the world are providing the answers that will help you to live longer, with a better quality of life. Hope is being turned into concrete benefits, even for people whose cancers have spread.

10

Genetic background to bowel cancer

Many people with colorectal cancer have a recurrence after surgery, so that there is a tremendous need for better prevention and treatment. Most colon cancers arise spontaneously, with no obvious inherited link. Eighty per cent of cases arise in people older than 65. However, inheriting, as Jacob did (see p. xi), a particular single gene defect among the 50,000 genes we possess can give us a 100 per cent risk of bowel cancer. People with these mutations belong to one of two types of family – those with familial adenomatous polyposis (FAP) and those with heritable non-polyposis colon cancer (HNPCC).

Cancer doesn't arise out of the blue, in a single physical change. The process of developing an invasive colorectal cancer happens in stages, one after the other, over many years. Patients who have the FAP mutation can develop in their teenage years from 500 to 5,000 benign tumours (polyps), which are mostly small. Some of them enlarge, and eventually one of these larger polyps becomes cancerous. The process takes 15 to 20 years, so that they develop cancer when they are aged between 30 and 40. In 'sporadic' cancer arising in people with no known relatives with the disease, there is no obvious early change in the bowel wall. This type of cancer also develops from a pre-cancerous stage, but it takes much longer to do so. This is why patients whose cancers come 'out of the blue' are usually much older (over 60) when their symptoms begin.

The transition from normal cell to cancerous cell involves a series of genes acting one after the other. I mention their names here not to confuse you with science, but to show how complex the process is, and also to show how much we already know about it. With this knowledge, new treatments can be developed to shut off the gene activity at each stage. So what follows here is meant to be encouraging, and not frightening. I am indebted to Professor Paraskeva (see p. 4) for the information.

The first stage is induced by the activity of 'APC/B-catenin' genes that convert normal colorectal wall cells into early adenomas, the first stage of polyps. The next stage, to late adenoma (now an obvious polyp on endoscopy), requires a mutation in the 'K-Ras' gene. Even at this stage, the tumour remains benign, and will only enlarge locally. A further mutation is needed, in genes called P53 and 18qLOH, before the cells spread beyond the gut, to become truly cancerous. It is vital to prevent that last stage. Obviously many research groups are now trying to find ways to 'switch off' all of these genes, to develop ways to prevent and to treat bowel cancer. They are also identifying other cancer-inducing genes as new targets for therapy.

Why do the genes 'switch on' in the first place? One well-established cause of cancerous change is chronic inflammation. Here again the book becomes technical, but please bear with me, as an understanding of the mechanisms of cancer induction in tissues helps you to cope with the treatment you will be asked to follow.

Cancers and chronic inflammation

The evidence that illnesses in which there is long-term ('chronic') inflammation can lead to cancer is strong. Defining 'inflammation' so that it can be understood by someone not trained in the biological sciences isn't easy, but please read on, because again it is important.

Inflammation is the body's reaction to a 'foreign' invader. This can be an attack by a germ or a protein that the body 'sees' as foreign. Occasionally this can be one of the body's own proteins that our immune system mistakenly recognizes as 'foreign'. Such illnesses are classified as 'auto-immune' diseases. They can affect the joints as in rheumatoid arthritis, or the thyroid gland, as in several forms of underactive or overactive thyroid disease, or the bowel wall, as in ulcerative colitis and Crohn's disease (see pp. 32–5). The development of colonic polyps can be looked upon as a form of inflammation.

Patients with ulcerative colitis and intestinal polyps are much more likely than normal to develop colon cancer. Schistosomiasis, a tropical disease in which an infection causes intense inflammation in the bladder, leads to bladder cancer. Recurrent prostatitis (the result of repeated prostate infections) may lead to prostate cancer. There are similar links between bronchitis and lung cancer; oesophagitis (heartburn due to acid regurgitation into the gullet) and oesophageal cancer; gastritis (inflammation of the stomach wall) and stomach cancer; and the virus infections hepatitis B and C and liver cancer.

Common to all of them are chronic immune alteration and inflammation.

In technical terms, in chronic inflammation the immune system switches from one type of reaction to another. There are two types of immune reaction – so named after the type of lymphocyte (a form of white blood cell) that the body uses to contain the inflammation. Normally they are in balance, working together to protect the body.

The technical names for these two types of immune response are cell-mediated (Th-1) and humoral-mediated (Th-2). The 'Th' stands for *thymocyte*, a type of white blood cell (a lymphocyte) that has been 'activated' by passing through the thymus gland inside the chest. The Th-1 response marshals the different white blood cells to any site of inflammation or infection, where they seek out the intruder and destroy it. The Th-2 response mobilizes the antibodies and other defensive chemical systems that fix on to the surface of the intruding foreign proteins and disrupt them.

Normally, the two systems work in tandem. However, chronic inflammation that is not overcome eventually leads to suppression of cell-mediated immunity. The Th-1 response dies away, leaving the Th-2 response in control by itself. The Th-2 response on its own stimulates the formation of new blood vessels around the affected site. If there is a cancerous change there, these blood vessels can carry off the cancer cells to distant parts of the body, where they can 'seed' and grow.

This production of new blood vessels (it's called *angiogenesis*) is present before the dramatic changes of cancer appear in the cells, and it can be reversed at this stage by stimulating the immune system in the right way. One way this can be done is to use drugs like aspirin.

How aspirin helps

Aspirin helps in several ways. First, it blocks the process of inflammation. Second, it stops angiogenesis. Third, it may even block the signals that the Th-2 chemical releases that lead to the initiation of the cancerous change.

This is not just theory. The first hint that aspirin and drugs like it such as non-steroidal anti-inflammatory drugs (NSAIDs) may be useful in colorectal cancer arose when patients with multiple polyps, and who were under regular observation to ensure that they were not turning cancerous, were given sulindac, an NSAID, for pain relief for other illnesses, such as arthritis. By chance it was found that their polyps shrank and some even disappeared. When the sulindac was stopped, the polyps recurred. Professor Paraskeva suggested that NSAIDs might work by causing the polyp (pre-tumour) cells to 'commit suicide'.

His group then found that regular users of aspirin for pain and inflammation (mainly for such conditions as arthritis) have half the normal risk of developing bowel cancer. They also have fewer benign tumours (adenomas) in their bowel wall. Professor Paraskeva explained how this happens.

How aspirin blocks COX

Aspirin blocks the action of an enzyme, found in all cells, called cyclo-oxidase, or COX. The main function of COX is to produce in the body a series of substances called prostaglandins (PGs) which are active in inflammation. There are two forms of COX. The first, COX-1, is produced by normal cells and protects the stomach wall against acid. COX-2 is not present in most normal cells and not present in the normal colon. But colon cancer cells and pre-malignant adenoma cells do produce large amounts of COX-2.

The consequent high PG levels increase cell growth, prevent the abnormal cells from dying off, increase their ability to spread within the tissues around them, and induce angiogenesis. All these properties together mean that the cells become more invasive within the bowel wall, and spread to other parts of the body. The rise in blood supply from the excess blood vessels helps tumours to grow and become more aggressive.

Aspirin blocks both the high COX-2 activity and the normal COX-1 activity. Its ability to prevent cancer is in part due to the COX-2 effect. Professor Paraskeva was in no doubt that when the risks of taking aspirin (a few people may suffer stomach bleeds) are outweighed by its advantages, then it should be given. He does not, though, recommend that the general public should take it routinely.

Aspirin and 'cell suicide'

Aspirin may even have another card to play in cancer. All our cells in every tissue are programmed to 'commit suicide' at the appropriate time in development or when something goes wrong.

The technical word for this is *apoptosis*. Professor Paraskeva used the example of cells in a tadpole tail, which must commit suicide to allow the creature to become a frog. In human development, cells in the webbing between fingers also undergo apoptosis. Every second, about 10 million cells die naturally from skin, blood cells and the colon as part of normal tissue turnover. They need to be continuously replaced by cell division. Each tissue must not continue to grow beyond what is necessary.

So we all possess genes that induce apoptosis. Professor Paraskeva proposed that some of the genes that are defective in people who inherit colorectal cancer are just such genes. If they do not work correctly, then cells no longer commit suicide when they are at the end of their lifespan – and these are the cells in which cancers start. Salicylates like aspirin may well promote cancer cell apoptosis by reprogramming them to do so. Leaves fall off trees because the cells at their base commit suicide. This may well be one of the functions of salicylates in plants, and it is entirely possible that salicylate may well have a similar effect in animals, including us.

Summing-up

Although the precise mechanisms by which aspirin and other NSAIDs protect against cancer are unclear, they have been shown to possess several different properties that combine to do so. Their effects are:

1 to block tumour cell proliferation (their propensity to multiply out of control within the boundaries of their normal tissue sites);
2 that they induce apoptosis (the self-destruction, or suicide, of cancer cells);
3 that they prevent the 'migration' of tumour cells beyond their normal limits to distant organs;
4 that they may even prevent cells from becoming cancerous in the first place by mechanisms that are still being studied.

Knowledge of all these mechanisms will surely help the researchers to develop novel treatments.

Salicylates and aspirin-like drugs are only the beginning, and no one is suggesting that they are a total cure. There are many other ways in which cancers can be attacked, and some of the drugs that have been developed from studying these anti-cancer pathways are already being researched. The future in the fight against colorectal cancer is bright.

11

Researching bowel cancer

One man in the forefront of this research is Professor John Burn, Clinical Director of the NHS Northern Genetics Service and Medical Director of the University of Newcastle upon Tyne Institute of Human Genetics. He, too, spoke at the seminal meeting in November 2003, which I mentioned on p. 4. He described his group's research projects in familial bowel cancer.

The CAPP1 trial

In 1993, Professor Burn and his colleagues launched CAPP1, the European Concerted Action on Polyp Prevention. It is now called the Colorectal Adenoma/Carcinoma Prevention Programme (also CAPP). Carriers of familial adenomatous polyposis (FAP) were recruited to a randomized placebo-controlled trial of 600 milligrams of aspirin and/or 30 grams of resistant starch. (Resistant starch is starch that is not digested until it reaches the large bowel, so it is a useful 'bulking agent' that might speed up transit of the contents of the large bowel.) In other words, some of the people in the trial took the aspirin, some the starch, some both, and some neither.

The background to CAPP1 was that there had been substantial evidence from population studies that these two treatments might prevent the development of adenomatous polyps, the precursor of colorectal cancer. Some 206 FAP carriers received treatment. By October 2003, completed data on 133 subjects followed for at least one year had been analysed. Neither the aspirin nor the starch had significantly reduced polyp numbers, as assessed by the endoscopist at the time of the examinations or by an independent expert reviewing videos of endoscopy appearances without knowledge of the patients or their previous polyp status. However, the difference in the largest polyp measurement was impressive. The placebo groups had bigger polyps than the aspirin-receiving groups. After more than a year, the biggest impact was in the aspirin-starch group. The polyps were half the size in the aspirin group, a result very encouraging for an effect on cancer.

Biopsies from the bowel wall of the trial subjects showed that the two different treatments had different effects on the microscopic appearance, one changing the length of the 'crypts' (folds in the lining of the bowel) and the other making the cells within the crypts more active. The changes both strongly suggest that the two drugs protect against cancer, but with different modes of action. Aspirin may act later in the evolution of bowel cancer than starch, by preventing progression of small adenomata.

Professor Burn stressed that these results are not simply relevant to FAP carriers. They are an ideal study group, he said, because they share their genetic defect with the majority of people who develop sporadic colorectal cancers. Any protective effect in FAP is likely to have general relevance to the rest of the population.

His team is now conducting CAPP2. This is testing aspirin and resistant starch in carriers of the other main inherited bowel cancer, hereditary non-polyposis colon cancer (HNPCC). By the end of 2003, more than 688 gene carriers of HNPCC had been entered into the study in 38 centres worldwide. The study is planned and supported by the new International Society for Gastrointestinal Hereditary Tumours – InSiGHT. This is a vital organization for bowel cancer sufferers, as it is through InSiGHT that most of the best research is co-ordinated. The work on aspirin and starch is only part of many other trials that InSiGHT is undertaking.

To be sure of getting the fastest results, Professor Burn's trials have had to concentrate on families with a known high risk of bowel cancer. However, he emphasizes that it is mainly an environmental issue, and not a genetic one. Between 75 and 80 per cent of bowel cancers arising before the age of 65 are potentially avoidable. If we can detect and treat them before they reach the stage of cancer, then this will be a huge benefit.

Today, of the young people with thousands of polypi in the colon, all will die in relatively early middle age if the colon is not removed. Recently we have been able to identify the carriers in the families, but as yet we still have to remove their colons. It would be good, though, to keep them from surgery being their only option.

A typical sufferer described by Professor Burn is John, a young man whose mother had had her colon and rectum removed (a *pan-proctocolectomy*) and had three children. Two of them are cancer gene carriers. One side effect of her gene problem is the growth of *osteomas* – benign bony lumps that grow anywhere in the body.

John had two bony bumps on his forehead, so that it was obvious to the Professor, without needing to test him, that he was one of the carriers. John knew this, too, and like all people who carry the genes, is highly motivated to help himself. They know why the cancers happen and are already in a follow-up programme, so they are happy to take part in well-run trials involving lifestyle changes and drugs for prevention or treatment.

Another of Professor Burn's patients is Stephen, who has a condition called Lynch syndrome, inherited from both his father and mother. Thirteen of his family members have cancer. It is due to a single gene mutation.

During studies of volunteers with pre-cancerous conditions of the colon, to see an actual change during the follow-up is relatively rare. Of the 500-plus colonoscopies in the CAPP2 study, the researchers have now observed only 50 new 'events' (i.e. areas in which there is evidence of a cancerous change). One hundred are needed to be able to calculate whether or not the drugs are working, so that setting up the trial and following it through is a long and slow process. Proposed in 1994, it was 1998 before EU and industrial funds were in place, and only in 1999 was it given ethical clearance to start. In 2002, the MRC awarded £2 million towards its costs. Getting a proposed trial, even in urgent subjects like cancer prevention, past the ethicists is now 'a nightmare', according to Professor Burn. Let's hope that things speed up in the next few years.

Some other anti-inflammatory drugs

Aspirin is not the only anti-inflammatory drug to be used in colon cancer prevention trials. On high doses of the new type of COX-2 blocker, celecoxib, there was a reduction in polyps. Sulindac, an older NSAID, will suppress polyps but may not suppress cancer: a case of cancer has developed in a bowel that showed a reduction in numbers of polyps on sulindac, and Drs Giardiello and Winde, who reported it, concluded that sulindac was of no benefit. Gunther Winde, one of these authors, has also reported on one patient who developed very rapidly growing rectal cancer while using sulindac suppositories. It may be that the aspirin action is specific to aspirin alone, and not a property shared by other anti-inflammatory drugs.

Research for the future

The research is going on apace. The British Familial Cancer Record organization is collecting DNA from cancer centres to determine the best way to focus on genetics to develop new treatments. By October 2003 it had received the medical and pathology reports of 274 cancers, 66 of which developed despite being on surveillance. InSiGHT is now the society to which all clinicians and researchers in bowel tumours belong. Its ability to communicate freely among all the research groups will surely greatly improve our knowledge of the disease and how to prevent and manage it.

Where does the research go from here? The results for aspirin so far suggest that it has the potential to substantially reduce numbers of colorectal cancers. However, this can only be proven by appropriately designed randomized controlled trials (RCTs), which must include thousands of people randomly assigned to be treated over many years with the appropriate doses of drugs or placebo, with neither the subject nor the doctor supervising the trial knowing whether or not the patient is on the active drug. The same strictures apply to research into any new drug to prevent colorectal cancer, whether anti-inflammatory or with another mode of action. More RCTs are therefore urgently needed to test our current theories of cancer initiation and spread.

The practicalities of conducting RCTs are far-reaching. Substantial investments of time and money are required and results take many years to obtain. On the evidence so far, we have already reached the point where such investments are required. For aspirin, in fact, there is good evidence that it may also reduce the risk of other cancers such as ovarian cancer and cancers of the stomach and oesophagus. In May 2004, breast cancer was added to this list.

Drawbacks of aspirin

There are two drawbacks to aspirin. One is that it has undesirable effects, such as irritation to the stomach wall, that may cause bleeding. So it should only be used when the benefits obviously outweigh its risks. The other is that it is very cheap and widely available over the pharmacy and supermarket counter. That raises the danger that far too many people may take it regularly without understanding its risks. If you are considering taking it, please discuss it with your doctor, and don't just start doing so on the basis that it may help you. If you do start to take it, always let your doctor know. There are some prescription drugs (such as warfarin for heart problems) that need to be taken with care, or not at all, if you are also taking aspirin. In any case, aspirin must only be used as a complement to, and not a competitor against, other prescribed treatments and lifestyle improvements.

Actually, advice on lifestyle improvements usually falls on stony ground. In many years of trials of diets versus drugs, Professor Peter Elwood, of the University of Wales, has found that intensive advice to increase fruit and vegetable intake, followed up with proper zeal, has little effect. Professor Elwood's work has concentrated on the lifestyles of older men in the Caerphilly area: they were most reluctant to change their poor eating habits. Perhaps men and women who know that they are at high risk of developing colorectal cancer are better motivated to do so.

12

When you have advanced bowel cancer

Unfortunately, around a third of people with colorectal cancer are found, at the first examination, to have tumours that have already spread beyond the bowel. They are in Dukes' stages C and D. This means that simply removing the tumour won't cure the disease. Something must be done to try to eliminate, or at least substantially reduce, the tumour mass – not just in the bowel, but elsewhere. That usually means using radiotherapy and chemotherapy. This chapter concentrates on what is on offer in British colorectal cancer centres.

If you have already visited one of these centres, you will know how very well the staff and the patients get on. They are places of caring and friendship, where the staff in all departments are very special and have a deep understanding of the fears and stresses that you, as a cancer patient, must feel. They also have a good idea of what is ahead of you, and will make it as bearable and pleasant as they know how. So if your doctor is sending you to a unit like this, please feel confident that you will be received very well, and that you will get the very best of attention and treatment. It is important not just for your peace of mind, but also for your survival, that you feel that the treatment is about making you better.

Once the full extent of your cancer spread is known, your surgical team will discuss the options for treatment with the *oncologists*, the cancer specialists. Their aim is still, if possible, to find a way of removing so much of your cancer that you are in effect 'cured'. In other words, that your cancer is under control and can be expected not to recur in a dangerous way, perhaps for many years. Even if that doesn't seem possible, there are still treatments designed to reduce the cancer load so much that your life will be extended for many months or even years, and that the quality of your life will be sustained.

The choices facing you and your doctors encompass further surgery, radiotherapy and chemotherapy. We will take them in turn, although in fact many people with advanced colorectal cancer will be offered a combination of some or all of them.

Surgery for secondary growths
(secondaries or metastases)

Cancers arising in the colon or rectum naturally spread towards the liver. It is common for surgeons to find, as they are removing bowel cancers, that there are one or more secondary deposits of cancer (*metastases*) in the substance of the liver. In the past, that was the sign that the cancer could not be removed, and the abdomen would be closed up again. The option then was for the patient to receive chemotherapy (which will be described later in this chapter), or radiotherapy, or be left without anti-cancer treatment of any sort. Much depended on how fit the patient was to withstand the treatment on offer at the time.

Today, surgeons are much more likely to try to remove the part, or parts, of the liver containing the tumours. If they can all be removed, the patient still has a chance of cure, and at least has a good possibility of surviving longer and in a healthier state. Here is a quote from Dr G. S. Gazelle and his colleagues, who reviewed the effectiveness of removal of liver secondaries (*hepatic metastasectomy*) in *Annals of Surgery* in 2003 (Gazelle and colleagues, 2003, pp. 544–55): 'There is substantial evidence that resection of liver metastases can result in long-term survival in some patients.'

They found that removing up to six metastases and with one repeat operation to remove other metastases six months later, the patients gained, on average, 2.63 extra 'quality-adjusted life years'(QALYs). QALYs are a measure not just of extra survival, but also of survival in a good physical state. The extra years shortened as the numbers of metastases removed increased, but the improvement in life for the patients operated upon was such that the surgeons advised their American colleagues that 'more aggressive approaches are preferred to less aggressive approaches' to liver metastases in bowel cancer. They encourage surgeons to consider resection for all patients whose metastases can be removed.

That message has been taken a stage further. For some people the only answer is to remove the whole liver and give them a transplant. Many studies of this treatment rate the five-year survival for people who have had total liver removal and transplant for colorectal cancer as between 20 and 45 per cent. However, for many people, their cancers are too advanced at diagnosis for them to be able to survive the operation. The cancer researchers therefore turned to trying to reduce the total size of the cancer mass in the liver before tackling the liver metastases. The most effective way to do this is to give the patients chemotherapy first.

If you are selected for this treatment, you have to be truly a *patient* in all senses, because it usually takes between five and ten months of chemotherapy before the operation can be performed. Singapore surgeon S. Y. Ong reviewed the trials of this treatment in March 2003 (Ong, 2003, pp. 205–11). He showed that up to 40 per cent of people who started on chemotherapy with no chance of a transplant were so improved by it that they were able to undergo it. Between 30 and 60 per cent of them were still alive and well five years later. Many of them have relapses confined to the liver, but they can be treated a second time, with the same good results. 'In carefully selected patients,' Ong writes, 'neoadjuvant chemotherapy may be able to downstage the disease adequately for curative resection.'

Chemotherapy

The term *neoadjuvant chemotherapy* needs to be explained, and to do that we need to know a little of the science behind the different aspects of chemotherapy and the drugs we use.

Chemotherapy is the name applied to the use of drugs to kill cancer cells. Specifically they are *cytotoxic* agents – agents that poison cells. They are classified into five main groups, the details of which are outside the scope of this book, but which comprise the alkylating agents, topoisomerase 1 inhibitors, cytotoxic antibiotics, antimetabolites and the vinca alkaloids. Although they act on different processes inside cancer cells to stop them increasing in number and spreading, they share one big problem.

That is, they attack cells when they are in the process of dividing (the way in which they increase in number). They kill cancer cells more readily than they kill normal cells because cancer cells are beyond the body's natural control systems and are dividing faster than normal cells. However, cells that normally replicate themselves very quickly are also affected by cytotoxic agents, so that they can slow down the production of new blood cells in the bone marrow, they can affect the lining cells of the stomach and intestine, and they shut down the cells in the hair roots.

That's why the main side effects of chemotherapy are anaemia and low white blood cell counts, nausea, and loss of hair. While you are on chemotherapy, therefore, you will have regular blood counts, and may also be given drugs to ease your nausea. A fall in blood count may not mean you need to stop treatment, but you may have to have transfusions before your next dose. As for the loss of hair, some people try to prevent it or minimize it by wearing ice bags on the head in the hours after their chemotherapy dose, but there is little good evidence that it works. Happily, the hair grows back in time.

The decisions on what to give as chemotherapy to people with advanced colorectal cancer are now guided in Britain by the National Institute for Clinical Excellence (NICE), whose experts have reviewed the many clinical trials of the various drugs. Put briefly, there are two main options for the first-line treatment for colorectal cancer that has spread beyond the bowel.

One is the combination of the 'antimetabolite' fluorouracil, combined with folinic acid. It is given intravenously. It is unusual for fluorouracil to produce severe side effects, although there are reports of bone marrow suppression (of both red cells and white cells) and of inflammation of the mouth (*mucositis*). Given for long periods it can cause the skin of the hands and feet to peel off. This is called hand-foot syndrome, and is unpleasant, but recovers as the drug is withdrawn.

Raltitrexed (Tomudex, technically a 'thymydilate synthase inhibitor') may be given intravenously when fluorouracil can't be used (perhaps because of a previous reaction to it). As with fluorouracil, most patients tolerate raltitrexed well, though some react with nausea and diarrhoea, and some with bone marrow suppression.

Another antimetabolite, capecitabine, has the advantage over the other antimetabolites by being given by mouth, in a pill. This allows it to be given as a treatment at home, rather than in the clinic. It gives the patient an extra boost to be able to treat himself or herself at home under the supervision of the specialist nurse, which is a partnership that is much valued by both. Once digested, it is turned into fluorouracil in the body, so its effects and side effects are similar. However, recent reports (Gerbrecht, 2003, pp. 161–7) warn that the hand-foot syndrome is perhaps more common on capecitabine than on injected fluorouracil. Nurses and patients need to be warned about its development.

Tegafur (Uftoral) is a similar oral drug that is converted into

87

fluorouracil in the body: it is usually given with another drug, calcium folinate.

In 2003, NICE gave its official guidance on which drugs or combinations should be used in advanced bowel cancer. It advised that fluorouracil and folinic acid, or capecitabine, or tegafur with uracil, be the options for first-line treatment for metastatic colorectal cancer.

There are two other drugs commonly used in advanced colorectal cancer: oxaliplatin and irinotecan. Oxaliplatin (Eloxatin) is a platinum compound, an alkylating agent, given by injection. Irinotecan (Campto) is also given by injection. They are both licensed by the European authorities to be given alongside fluorouracil and folinic acid for first-line treatment of colorectal cancer that has metastasized. NICE, however, does not recommend this. Instead it advises that the combination of oxaliplatin and fluorouracil/folinic acid should be given only to patients with liver metastases that could be removed surgically after treatment. This is the *neoadjuvant chemotherapy* described by Dr Ong. Many cancer specialists would disagree with this decision by NICE, and will continue to prescribe the combination in specific cases even though they do not plan liver surgery. It is hard to disagree with them.

NICE recommends that irinotecan treatment on its own be given to patients failing to respond to the usual fluorouracil-containing treatments. It does not recommend raltitrexed for general use yet, preferring that it should still be confined to trials. However, raltitrexed is available for use in Britain, and is yet another option for patients for whom other treatments have been less than successful.

Managing the side effects

A piece on chemotherapy would not be complete without describing ways to minimize the side effects of the drugs used. The main side effects for anti-colorectal cancer drugs are mucositis and nausea and vomiting.

The best way to deal with mucositis is to prevent it if possible, with good mouth care. That involves rinsing the mouth regularly and cleaning the teeth with a soft brush two to three times daily. Sucking ice 'chips' during infusions of fluorouracil can help a lot. If you have developed a sore mouth, salt water (saline) mouthwashes should be used regularly. Mucositis does die down, but it must be treated with good hygiene, as otherwise it can be a source of severe infection at a time when you are very vulnerable.

Nausea and vomiting can be 'acute' in that it occurs soon after treatment starts, or 'delayed' in that it starts more than 24 hours later. It can also be 'anticipatory', starting actually before the infusion begins. According to the authors of the 2004 edition of the *British National Formulary* (the 'bible' for prescribing doctors, produced by the British Medical Association and the Royal Pharmaceutical Society), the people most susceptible to nausea and vomiting as a response to cytotoxic drugs are women, people under 50, those with anxiety, and people who are prone to motion sickness (both carsickness and seasickness). Susceptibility to nausea becomes worse as you have repeated doses of the drug.

However, even if these claims regarding susceptibilty are correct, it is clear that some drugs are more likely to cause nausea and sickness than others. Fluorouracil, for example, is classified in the 'mild' group of emetic drugs. Cisplatin is in the 'highly emetogenic' (sickness-inducing) group.

To prevent acute sickness, in the first instance most people are given either domperidone or metoclopramide, two well-established anti-emetic drugs. Dexamethasone (a steroid) or lorazepam (a tranquillizer) may be added if domperidone or metoclopramide do not work. Just as effective may be drugs called 5HT3 blockers. They include granisetron, ondansetron and tropisetron. They are probably better than the other anti-emetics if the nausea and vomiting are expected to be severe.

Dexamethasone is the best drug to prevent the delayed nausea: it is often given with metoclopramide or prochlorperazine. As for preventing the anticipatory sickness, reassurance and relaxation are probably the most helpful treatment. However, they are not always possible to accept, understandably, in the hours before a dose of chemotherapy, so that lorazepam may be a good choice here. It is not only a good treatment for anxiety, it also makes you sleepy and so helps you to forget the treatment period. In fact, it often leaves you with amnesia for the period around the treatment.

Radiotherapy

Radiation therapy is used mainly for rectal cancer. It is given mainly just before surgery to try to 'shrink' tumours so that they can be totally removed more easily and with the least disturbance to the patient. In particular, radiation before surgery can help the surgeon operating on a rectal cancer to preserve the anal sphincter – the muscle that controls defaecation. This can obviously be a big bonus to the patient who might otherwise be incontinent or need a colostomy.

In 2003, Dr B. Glimelius and colleagues of Uppsala, Sweden, reviewed the results of such radiation therapy from articles encompassing 25,351 patients, and compared them with similar results published in 1996. They showed that the results of rectal cancer surgery have improved in the last eight years. The numbers of failures within five years of the surgery fell from 28 per cent to 10–15 per cent. Giving pre-operative radiation lowers the risk of failure by between 50 and 70 per cent, and improves long-term survival by about 10 per cent.

Dr Glimelius wrote that there is some indication that more people survive for longer if they are given both radiation therapy and chemotherapy after the operation. Radiation can be used like neoadjunctive chemotherapy in patients with rectal cancers, to reduce inoperable tumours into operable ones. Even if the cancer is not turned into an operable one, radiotherapy will often relieve the more severe symptoms of the disease, such as obstruction and tenesmus.

Radiation therapy is particularly well suited to cancers right at the end of the digestive tract – the anal skin. Cure rates for such cancers are as high for radiation with or without chemotherapy as for surgery to remove them (Newlin and colleagues, 2004, pp. 55–62).

13

Some special cases – the older and the younger patient

Thankfully, we can now do something for every person with colorectal cancer, regardless of their age. In the past, older patients might have been denied anti-cancer treatment because they were 'too old'. In younger people, the cancer might have been missed altogether 'because young people don't get colon cancer'. Thanks to greater understanding and recognition of the disease, proper diagnosis and treatment can go a long way towards improving survival.

The older patient

In the past, age was a barrier to treatment for colorectal cancer. If you were old and had advanced colorectal cancer, you were given 'palliative therapy' (i.e. nursed and cared for, but with no sense that the tumour was being treated). It was often just a case of transferring the patient to a terminal care ward or, in more recent times, a hospice. This was thought to be a kindness, because older people were thought too frail to be able to tolerate either surgery or chemotherapy.

That has changed, and there is plenty of evidence now that even at the age of 80 men and women with colorectal cancers benefit just as much from curative surgery or from chemotherapy for metastatic cancer as younger adults (Au and colleagues, 2003, pp. 165–71). However, there are some aspects of the treatment with which care must be taken. For example, fluorouracil seems to cause more toxic side effects (see Chapter 12) in the old than in the young. P. C. Enzinger and R. J. Mayer wrote in April 2004 that, 'Adjuvant therapy for both colon and rectal cancer is underutilized in elderly patients, despite such lifesaving treatments resulting in similar survival prolongation as well as toxicity profiles, as in their younger counterparts' (Enzinger and Mayer, 2004, pp. 206–19).

Treating elderly patients for their colorectal cancers is even cost-effective, according to New York surgeon M. J. Matasar and his colleagues. They wrote in 2004 that surgeons are operating on the elderly with greater frequency, less operative mortality, and greater success. Their five-year survival following potentially curative surgery has risen from 50 per cent to 67 per cent.

Matasar's group state that when using fluorouracil along with surgery, 71 per cent of the elderly survive for five years or more, compared with 64 per cent who have surgery alone. In their study, adding irinotecan adds a further two months of survival over fluorouracil alone. These survival figures are astonishing, particularly considering that many of the elderly would have a life expectancy of around five years anyway, regardless of whether or not they have cancer. The benefits of adding the other newer drugs are not yet clear.

The message from these groups is that your age doesn't matter as to whether you are offered treatment for, or survive, colorectal cancer. Your fitness and your disease stage does matter, but whatever your age you should be given the appropriate surgery, chemotherapy and radiation therapy. You will have just as much chance of surviving them as people much younger than you.

The younger patient

Although colorectal cancer is mainly a disease of older people, it does arise in many people under 40. Colorectal cancer in these younger adults is more aggressive than in older people, in that when they present for the first time to their doctors with symptoms, it is often already at a late stage. The tumours look more aggressive, too, when examined under the microscope. However, if the cancer is caught early, in Dukes's stage A, then their five-year survival is much better than that of older people.

The researchers who made this review stressed that family doctors and other health care providers should be alert to the possibilities of colorectal cancer in younger adults, particularly because there are now 'excellent' ways of treating it.

Screening

This raises the subject of screening our apparently healthy population for colorectal cancer, because it is the only way many of these cancers in younger people will be detected in time to ensure a cure.

How that can be afforded is one question, and how it can be accomplished is another. We need a cheap test that will detect bowel cancer early, and the one that immediately springs to mind is the faecal occult blood test. It has been shown in communities in which this was wisely utilized that it detected early cancers with enough frequency to lower death rates from them. However, very few people, a small proportion of the population who need to be screened, will come for screening. To collect a sample of faeces is outside the normal experience of people, and most are unwilling to do it. It is different once people have symptoms that worry them, but we would like to catch the cancers before that stage.

If we could add flexible sigmoidoscopy (using a fibre-optic endoscope to examine the colorectal region, including the sigmoid colon) to the faecal blood test, this would increase the numbers of lives saved, but it would be costly. The recommendation in Britain is that all men and women should have faecal occult blood tests performed at age 50 or older, at least once. In people with relatives who have had bowel cancer at a younger age, the age limit should be scrapped and they should be monitored regularly.

The above is the ideal. Sadly, in all the efforts to get screening for bowel cancer started in Britain, the returns have been negligible. Very few have bothered to turn up for their check – far fewer, for example, than for breast screening. In the United States, since the mid-1990s everyone has been recommended to have a flexible sigmoidoscopy when they reach 50. If they are 'clear', then they are asked to have a repeat sigmoidoscopy every five years.

The *Journal of the American Medical Association* (*JAMA*) reported in 2003 the results of a massive study of 154,000 apparently healthy people aged 55 to 74 who were asked to undergo sigmoidoscopy. More than a thousand had pre-cancerous polyps or cancers: they were put into treatment programmes. Just as important, 11,500 people who were found to be free of any polyps or cancers at that first examination were asked to come back for a second sigmoidoscopy three years later.

Americans seem to be good at answering requests to come in to their doctors' offices for tests. Of the 11,500 asked to return, 9,317 actually did so – 80 per cent. Of them, 1,292 (14 per cent) had abnormal growths in their colons, 292 of which turned out to be cancerous. So, three years after a negative result for colorectal cancer, 3.1 per cent of them, now aged 58 to 77, had developed it.

The inevitable conclusion is for older people to have bowel examinations more often than is now the case.

Is it feasible, and for that matter affordable, to ask the whole population to have regular examinations for bowel cancer so as to detect the few who are developing it? That is the current debate. A 'hit rate' of 3.1 per cent is high for any mass screening, and could well be worthwhile in saving many lives. However, current British attitudes to screening for bowel diseases will have to change to make it happen. I guess that will take time. Perhaps the best argument I can put forward is that since I started to research the material for this book, I decided to have a flexible sigmoidoscopy myself. Thankfully, I'm clear.

14

The future – new targets for treatment

Where can we go from here? For the scientists, the answer is clear – inside the cancer cell molecules. Now that we understand the molecular basis for the cancer change in cells, we can try to reverse or block the process that initiates or perpetuates the change. If that is achievable, the cancer cells will stop growing and will be eliminated, with a 'magic bullet' that will hit them, but at the same time spare all other, normal, cells.

One example of this is the finding of large amounts of the substance epidermal growth factor (EGF) in tumour tissues. Along with that, on the surface of the cancer cells the normal numbers of 'receptors' for EGF are very greatly multiplied, so that the cells can receive EGF and be stimulated to grow far faster than they would otherwise do. Blocking the EGF receptor has already produced benefits in human beings with cancer. A system called 'monoclonal antibodies' is used to produce exactly the right molecule to fit the patient's own unique tumour.

Another approach has been to create a blocker to the receptor of another growth factor, vascular growth factor (VGF). This system, too, depends on the creation of a monoclonal antibody (this one has a name, bevacizumab). The effect of such drugs is to shut down the ability of the tumour cells to create new blood vessels around them, literally starving the tumour cells to death. Aspirin-like drugs such as COX-2 inhibitors are also under study, as mentioned earlier.

We are still in the early stages of being able to conquer colorectal cancer, but the figures for cure and long-term increase in life expectancy have been rising steadily over the last ten years. The next ten years will see an even bigger jump in detection and cures of this disease.

References

Annals of Internal Medicine, vol. 139, 2003, pp. 51–5, 56–70.

Au, H. J., and colleagues, *Clinical Colorectal Cancer*, vol. 3, November 2003, pp. 165–71.

British Medical Journal, vol. 327, August 2003.

Enzinger, P. C., and Mayer, R. J., *Seminars in Oncology*, vol. 31, April 2004, pp. 206–19.

Gazelle, G. S., and colleagues, *Annals of Surgery*, vol. 237, 2003, pp. 544–55.

Gerbrecht, B. M., *Cancer Nursing*, vol. 26, April 2003, pp. 161–7.

Gumovsky-Reicher, S., and colleagues, *MedGenMed*, vol. 5, 10 January 2003, p. 16.

Kmietowicz, Zosia, *British Medical Journal*, vol. 328, 7 February 2004, p. 303.

Leung, Ka Lau, and colleagues, *Lancet*, vol. 363, 10 April 2004, pp. 1187–92.

Matasar M. J., and colleagues, 'Management of colorectal cancer in elderly patients: focus on the cost of chemotherapy', *Drugs and Aging*, vol. 21, no. 2, 2004, pp. 113–33.

Newlin, H. E., and colleagues, *Surgical Oncology*, vol. 86, 1 May 2004, pp. 55–62.

Ong, S. Y., *Annals Academy of Medicine of Singapore*, vol. 32, 2003, pp. 205–11.

Peters, Ulrika, and colleagues, *Lancet*, vol. 361, May 2003, pp. 1491–5.

Sanders, D. S., and colleagues, 'Association of adult coeliac disease with irritable bowel syndrome: a case-control study in patients fulfilling ROME II criteria referred to secondary care', *Lancet*, vol. 358, December 2001, pp. 1504–8.

Scheidbach, H., and colleagues, *Minerva Chirurgica*, vol. 58, 2003, pp. 439–46.

Tekkis, P., and colleagues, *British Medical Journal*, vol. 327, August 2003, pp. 1196–9.

Thompson, M. R., and colleagues, *British Medical Journal*, vol. 327, August 2003, pp. 263–5.

Thompson, W. G., and colleagues, 'Functional bowel disorders and functional abdominal pain', *Gut*, vol. 45, 1999, pp. 1143–7.

Index

Alan *see* case studies
alcohol 3
alverine 63
anaemia 44
aspirin 3, 5–7, 75–8, 82–3
Atkins, Dr 2–3

barium studies 56
beta-carotene 12
Brooke, Professor Brian 58–9
Burn, Professor John 79–81

CAPP1/CAPP2 studies 79–81
case studies
  Alan 51–2
  Jacob x
  James 36–41
  Jane 45–7
  Jenny 10–11
  Lawrence 47–8
  Mary 41–5
  Polly 50–1
  Rachel 49–50
  Walter 48–9
CAT scans 56–7
celecoxib 81
cell suicide 76–7
chemotherapy 46, 86–8
  managing side effects of
    88–9
cholera 24
coeliac disease 63–6
colonoscopy 56
colpermine 63

constipation 20–1
Crohn, Dr Burrell 21
Crohn's disease xii, 1, 21,
  32–4
Cumming, Dr 59–60

depression 10
diarrhoea 21–35
diverticular disease 66–7
Dukes' staging 57, 84

E. coli 28
elderly 91–2
Elwood, Professor Peter 83
Entamoeba histolytica 29
Enzinger, Dr P. C. 91

familial adenomatous polyposis
  (FAP) xii, 1
fartometer 59–60
follow-up, importance of 71–2

Gazelle, Dr G. S. 85
genetics of bowel cancer 73–4
Giardiello, Dr 81
Glimelius, Dr B. 90
growth factors 95

Helicobacter pylori 6
hereditary non-polyposis
  colorectal cancer
  (HNPCC) xii, 1

inflammation in bowel cancer
  74–5